The PD Companion

Life With
PARKINSON'S

50 FACTS
M&RE

Life With
PARKINSON'S
50 FACTS
M&RE

Clinical Reviewer

Alberto J. Espay, MD, MSc, FAAN, FANA
*Professor of Neurology
Director and Endowed Chair
James J. and Joan A. Gardner Center for Parkinson's Disease
and Movement Disorders
University of Cincinnati Academic Health Center*

Dr. Alberto Espay is Director and Endowed Chair of the James J. and Joan A. Gardner Center for Parkinson's Disease and Movement Disorders at the University of Cincinnati. He has published over 300 research articles and 7 neurology textbooks, including *Common Movement Disorders Pitfalls*, which received the highly commended BMA Medical Book Award in 2013. With Parkinson's patient and advocate Benjamin Stecher, he co-wrote *Brain Fables, the Hidden History of Neurodegenerative Diseases and a Blueprint to Conquer Them*, selected by the Association of American Publishers for the PROSE Award honoring the best scholarly work in Neuroscience published in 2020. He has served as Chair of the Movement Disorders Section of the American Academy of Neurology, Associate Editor of Movement Disorders, and on the Executive Committee of the Parkinson Study Group. He currently serves the International Parkinson and Movement Disorders Society as Chair of the Task Force on Technology and as Secretary of its Pan-American Section. His research efforts have focused on the measurement of motor and behavioral phenomena in, and clinical trials for, Parkinson's disease as well as on the understanding and management of functional movement disorders. Dr. Espay has received numerous awards, including the Dean's Scholar in Clinical Research award, the Dystonia Coalition Career Development award, the NIH-funded K23 Career Development award, the Cincinnati Business Courier's Forty Under 40 award, the Health Care Hero award, the Patients' Choice and Compassionate Doctor awards, the Excellence in Mentoring award, and the Spanish Society of Neurology's Cotzias award. With colleagues at the University of Cincinnati, he recently launched the first biomarker study of aging (CCBPstudy.com), designed to match people with neurodegenerative disorders to available therapies from which they are most biologically suitable to benefit, regardless of clinical diagnoses.

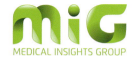

Disclaimer: This educational publication is intended to serve as an overview of topics related to Parkinson's disease. It is written for people with Parkinson's, caregivers, and others affected by the condition. The publisher, authors, and reviewer have taken care to ensure that the content is up-to-date, but as new information becomes available, changes in medical approaches become necessary. This material is for informational purposes only. It does not replace the advice or counsel of a doctor or health care professional. Readers should consult with and follow the advice of their doctor or health care provider. The publisher, authors, and reviewer disclaim responsibility for any liability, loss, injury, or damage incurred as a consequence, directly or indirectly, of the use and/or application of any content contained in this publication.

© Copyright 2022, Medical Insights Group, Inc. 125 Cabrini Boulevard, Floor 2, Suite A22, New York, NY 10033

Printed in the USA. All rights reserved, including the right of reproduction, in whole or in part, in any form.

Parkinson's Disease Today & Tomorrow

Parkinson's disease (PD) is not a single disease, but many. There are numerous genetic, biological, and environmental influences that render an individual vulnerable to developing PD. Each individual harbors a unique combination of these influences.

The approach to managing PD requires tailoring treatment to individual needs. Two types of tailoring in particular have become buzzwords of late: personalized medicine and precision medicine.

Personalized medicine is about optimizing symptomatic treatments and lifestyle changes to address the individual, symptom-specific source of difficulties. Symptoms result in part from deficiencies in certain neurotransmitters, and these deficiencies are very common across most people diagnosed with PD—common enough to allow PD to be diagnosed based on the symptoms with which they are associated. One very eloquent common denominator is dopamine deficiency. In a dopamine-deficient state, movements slow down, muscles stiffen, and a resting tremor may appear. Correcting dopamine levels with levodopa can normalize movements, lift the stiffness, and abolish the tremor. If an individual also has blood pressure fluctuations and depression, additional "personalized treatments" will be needed to optimize mobility, function, and ultimately quality of life.

Precision medicine is a different animal. Precision is about the biology in an individual, and is not necessarily concerned with the "average" of a population. We have gotten to know a lot about PD—the variably expressed, but ultimately single entity, ostensibly made up of many genetic, molecular, and toxic exposures whose common denominators we can diagnose at the bedside with a neurologic examination but for which we have no laboratory confirmation. But we know next to nothing about the PD of any particular individual. If we were to ever know what actually caused PD in a person, the therapeutic opportunity that opens will likely be of use to only the very few who shared the same exact biological type of PD—and no one else.

Until recently, most research into PD assumed that when a given abnormality is found in an affected person or family, such finding becomes a "piece of the overall puzzle" to explain PD in everyone. We are now recognizing that PD constitutes a unique puzzle in each person. Resolving that puzzle is the aspiration of precision medicine, already attained in other fields of medical practice.

The pages ahead are a testament to how far we can now get in personalizing the treatment (and overall support) of people with PD. I believe a future rendition of **Life With Parkinson's 50 Facts & More** *will ultimately share the first successes of true precision medicine.*

With my best wishes,

Alberto J. Espay, MD, MSc, FAAN, FANA

Life With
PARKINSON'S
**50 FACTS
M&RE**

Table of Contents

If you would like to purchase an additional copy of **The PD Companion** for a friend, caregiver, family member, or a person with PD, simply scan this QR code.

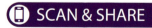

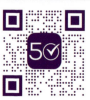

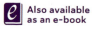

Introduction to the 50 Facts 9

SECTION 1: WHAT IS PARKINSON'S DISEASE? 13

What causes Parkinson's disease? 17
How common is Parkinson's disease? 17
Typical age at diagnosis 18
Are there factors that increase the risk for Parkinson's disease? 19
How is Parkinson's disease diagnosed? 22
What are motor symptoms? 23
    Resting tremor, bradykinesia, and stiffness 23
    Other motor symptoms 24
    Further evaluation & diagnosis 26
    Who can diagnose Parkinson's disease? 26
    Role of imaging 27
What are non-motor symptoms and complications? 28
    Psychiatric 29
    Sleep 32
    Pain 34
What is the goal of treating Parkinson's disease? 36
    The need to individualize treatment 36
    Lifestyle strategies 37

SECTION 2: PARKINSON'S DISEASE & TREATMENTS .. 41

Personal health literacy & Parkinson's 42
A Parkinson's Primer Approach: **Achieving PD Health Literacy** ... 43
Understanding the Mechanics of Parkinson's Disease 44
    The role of neurons in PD 44
    Signal transmissions 45
    Dopamine receptors 46
    The blood-brain barrier 47
    How is dopamine made? 48
    How is dopamine eliminated? 49
    Dopamine balance 50

SECTION 2 (CONT)

Understanding Treatment Approaches for Motor Symptoms With Medicine.. **52**
   3 ways to approach dopamine loss 52
   1-Treating low dopamine 53
      Levodopa 53
      Carbidopa 56
      Motor fluctuations 59
      "Off" episodes 60
      Overstimulation 62
   2-Providing a substitute for dopamine 64
      Dopamine agonists 64
   3-Slowing dopamine elimination 66
      MAO-B inhibitors 66
      COMT inhibitors 68
   Other medicines for treating motor symptoms 70

Understanding Treatment Approaches for Motor Symptoms (Devices & Surgery) **72**
   Intestinal levodopa infusion 73
   Deep brain stimulation 73
   Ablative surgery 74

Overview of Non-Motor Symptoms & Approaches **76**
   Cognitive symptoms 76
   Depression 78
   Anxiety 80
   PD psychosis 82
   Impulse control disorders 84
   Pseudobulbar affect 86
   Neurogenic orthostatic hypotension 88
   Sleep problems 90
   Pain 92
   Constipation 94
   Bladder issues 95
   Speech & voice problems 96
   Sialorrhea 98
   Sexual dysfunction 100

SECTION 3: ON THE ROAD—THE PD JOURNEY 103

- Pack a Positive Attitude for the Trip 105
- A Postcard From Frank C. Church: See yourself happy 106
- Mileposts: Frequently Asked Directions (FADs) 108
  - Me & My Parkinson's 108
    - PD & Me 108
    - PD & Family-Social Network 112
    - PD Health Care & Safety 118
    - My PD Life 124
    - PD & My Job 134
    - PD & My Finances 140
  - Partners & Caregivers 148
    - Preparing for a Caregiver Role 152
    - Appointments & Insurance 154
    - PD Medicine Management 156
  - Family, Friends, & Coworkers 160
    - How Can I Help? 160
    - Communication Tips 161
    - Supporting Our Colleague With PD 162
- *Frank's Circle of Words* 164

SECTION 4: THE FACES OF PARKINSON'S DISEASE ... 166

- Famous People With PD & Their Stories 167

APPENDICES 183

- **A.** PD Safety & Ease of Use: Changes for the Home 184
- **B.** PD Abbreviations & Acronyms 194
- **C.** Glossary & Index: PD Keywords & Definitions 196
- **D.** Index to Key Figures 210
- **E.** Parkinson's Resources 211
- **F.** References 212

"For everything this disease has taken, something with greater value has been given—sometimes just a marker that points me in a new direction that I might not otherwise have traveled.

So, sure, it may be 1 step forward and 2 steps back, but after a time with Parkinson's, I've learned that what is important is making that 1 step count; always looking up."

—Michael J. Fox

Life With
PARKINSON'S
50 FACTS
M&RE

INTRODUCTION

Life With Parkinson's 50 Facts & More is a valuable resource for readers on the Parkinson's disease (PD) journey. Whether you have just recently been diagnosed, are an experienced person with Parkinson's, or are in the crucial role of PD support, the following pages are chock-full of key learnings, facts, and explanations designed to both increase the reader's PD health literacy and to be referred to time and again as each Parkinson's path uniquely continues onward.

This resource provides a window into PD: what to expect, how to manage it, and how to continue living well with the disease. To that end, the reader will discover that each section's introduction comes with a list of important PD-related terms and concepts that are further discussed in that section. When each term is first used, it will be **listed in bold type**. Readers should not be intimidated by the language of Parkinson's. An important component of gaining control and understanding of PD's many challenges is gaining familiarity with what this new language will be in your life. These keywords and concepts are then matched with their definitions within the handy glossary at the very end of this reference guide. Anytime our readers are confronted with having to understand for the first time, or reacquaint themselves once more, with the many PD-related terms and concepts, they can refer back to the extensive glossary at the back of the book.

About 1 million adults in the United States have PD. It mainly affects people older than 50 years of age. **Living with PD requires a strong support system, so family, friends, and caregivers will have an important role on this journey.**

PD causes changes in your brain that make it harder to coordinate and control your movements. The symptoms you experience and how they affect you may be different than those experienced by others with PD. The most common characteristic symptoms of PD are called "motor symptoms," and include slow movement, tightness and stiffness in your muscles, and a resting tremor. These symptoms usually start on one side of the body, then move to both sides.

Although there is no cure for PD because it is not 1 disease and "a cure" can only be attained 1 individual at a time (in a "precision medicine" future), there are many treatments available to help manage your specific symptoms. Levodopa is the cornerstone of PD treatment. It helps increase dopamine levels in your brain to improve motor symptoms, which are largely caused by having too little dopamine. Treating PD can be challenging, especially as the disease progresses. You may end up needing higher doses of levodopa, additional medicines, or other lifestyle changes. **Fortunately, there are many medicines and other treatments available to you**.

You may also experience symptoms that do not affect your movement. These **"non-motor symptoms"** (sometimes referred to as "invisible symptoms") may include having trouble finding a word or multitasking; having episodes of anxiety, excessive sweating, or depression; experiencing blood pressure fluctuations or having sleep difficulties. After your diagnosis, you may realize that you had these non-motor symptoms for months or years before seeing a doctor. These symptoms can impact your life just as much as, or sometimes more than, your motor symptoms. Fortunately, these can be treated as well. **It is important to talk with your care team about your non-motor symptoms and how they can best be managed**.

Lastly, it is important to remember that PD is a lifelong journey and that symptoms, needs, and treatments will change over time. It can affect your everyday life and you will need new strategies to cope with these changes. Eventually, it may also be necessary to make changes to your home, mealtime routines, and travel so that you can continue to safely do the things you enjoy while **living well with your disease**.

"Happiness is not the absence of problems; it's the ability to deal with them."
—Steve Maraboli

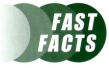

Considerable research is ongoing to further understand how PD affects your life and to investigate new treatment opportunities. These efforts are supported by numerous organizations, including the National Institutes of Health (ninds.nih.gov) and The Michael J. Fox Foundation for Parkinson's Research (michaeljfox.org).

In an effort to understand the subtypes of PD, several "biomarker discovery" programs have been created, with information available online for each of them.

Program	Website
The Parkinson's Progression Markers Initiative (PPMI)	michaeljfox.org/ppmi
The Luxembourg National Sleep Study	parkinson.lu
The Personalized Parkinson Project (PPP)	parkinsonopmaat.nl/en/study
The Cincinnati Cohort Biomarker Program (CCBP)	ccbpstudy.com

Keywords & Concepts Introduced in Section 1*

- Aggravators
- Anosmia
- Antioxidants
- Anxiety
- Atrophy
- Autonomic functions
- Bradykinesia
- Clinical trials
- Constipation
- DaTscan
- Davis Phinney Foundation for Parkinson's
- Delusions
- Depression
- Dopamine
- Dream enactment behaviors
- Drug-induced parkinsonism
- Dysphagia
- Dystonia
- Early-onset Parkinson's disease
- Environmental toxins
- Essential tremor
- Excessive daytime sleepiness (EDS)
- Facial masking
- Facilitators
- Freezing
- Freezing of gait
- Hallucinate
- Hallucinations
- Hypomimia
- Impulse control disorder (ICD)
- Inner tremor
- Insomnia
- Involuntary rhythmic motion
- Juvenile PD
- Magnetic resonance imaging (MRI)
- Micrographia
- Motor symptoms
- Movement disorder specialists
- Neurodegenerative condition
- Neurogenic orthostatic hypotension
- Neurologic
- Neurologist
- Neurons
- Neurotransmitter
- Nocturia
- Non-motor symptoms
- Parkinson's disease psychosis (PDP)
- Postural instability
- Postural reflexes
- Precision medicine
- Pseudobulbar affect (PBA)
- Resting tremor
- Rigidity
- Sialorrhea
- Stooped
- Substantia nigra
- Triggers

*Terms listed here are addressed in this section and can be found with their definitions in the Glossary (page 196).

SECTION 1: WHAT IS PARKINSON'S DISEASE?

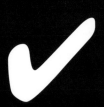

Parkinson's disease (**PD**) is a **neurodegenerative condition** that affects the brain. People with PD have trouble coordinating and controlling their movements, and can also have symptoms beyond movement disorders. Over time, PD can affect their ability to complete daily tasks. The symptoms affecting movement are called **motor symptoms**. Symptoms that do not affect movement can also occur. These are called **non-motor symptoms**.

PD is the second most common neurodegenerative disease.
The *most* common is Alzheimer's disease.

The body controls motion, in part, through a **neurotransmitter** called **dopamine**, within a region of the brain known as the **substantia nigra**. With PD, your brain function declines. Part of this decline involves a reduction of dopamine levels in the substantia nigra, which contributes to abnormal and uncontrolled movement, discussed in further detail in section 2.

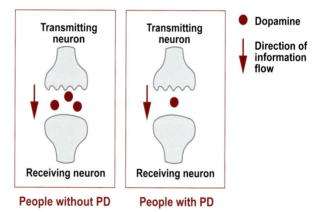

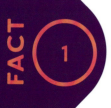

People with Parkinson's can have a good quality of life.

The substantia nigra is located near the middle of the brain and plays an important role in movement.

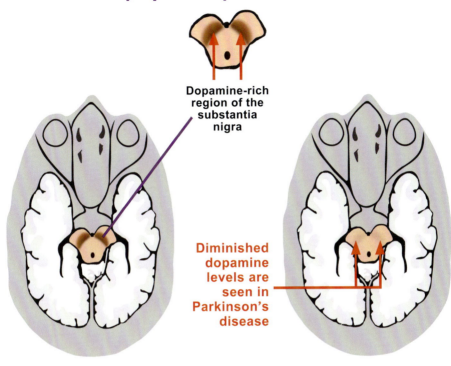

Dopamine-rich region of the substantia nigra

Diminished dopamine levels are seen in Parkinson's disease

People without PD

People with PD

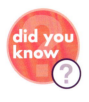

People who have Parkinson's disease experience a decline in their brain function due, in part, to a reduction of dopamine levels.

Life With **PARKINSON'S**

For research purposes, Parkinson's disease can be divided into 5 stages. They are applied in research so that participants in clinical trials can be grouped by similar levels of disability. Using stages in clinical care is not useful because each person's PD is different and many may never experience advanced "stages." Progression to a wheelchair is not predictable. **If you wish to know how researchers label each stage, here is a summary of those levels:**

Stage 1	Stage 2	Stage 3	Stage 4	Stage 5
Symptoms are minor and occur on one side of the body. You can perform all daily activities	Symptoms are worse and occur on both sides of the body. You can perform daily activities; however, it may be difficult. You will probably not experience any falls	Falls occur; however, you can live independently. Daily tasks, like dressing and eating, become challenging	Walking may require assistance. Symptoms are more severe. You are not able to live independently and you need help with daily activities	Symptoms are debilitating. You require a wheelchair or spend most of your time in bed. Nursing care is required. Disabling non-motor symptoms are also present

Symptoms of PD vary from person to person. Not everyone will experience every symptom. Symptoms may also progress differently for each individual.

The reality is that there is no single path that all people with PD follow. Rather, each individual is on their own unique journey, related in part to their unique genetics, biology, and risk factors. As a result, symptoms and their severity vary greatly from person to person.

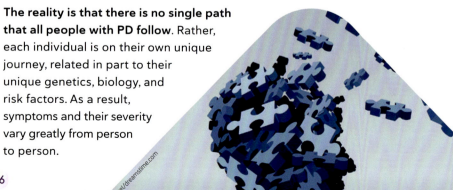

No 2 people with Parkinson's have the same exact symptoms.

2 FACT

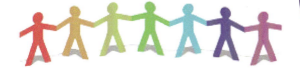

RobinOlimb/gettyimages.com

What causes Parkinson's disease?

There is no single cause that can explain PD for everyone affected with this disease. Some people have a genetic cause, whereas others may have developed Parkinson's as a result of being exposed to **environmental toxins**. **Other factors may work in combination:**

- Risk factors such as exposure to pesticides and use of well water could affect some more than others (page 19)
- Head trauma can also contribute to PD in those individuals with a biological susceptibility.

Each of these factors contributes to a distinct form of PD for each individual, but all of them lead to a decrease in dopamine availability in the substantia nigra, which causes problems with movement. **The reason why each person with PD does not make sufficient dopamine is unique to that individual.** Most research assumes that there are common causes to explain the disease. Researchers are now recognizing that this may not always be the case, and steps are being taken to individualize the approach—through a principle known as **precision medicine**—(page 3) to manage PD and tailor treatment to the unique causes of the disease in each individual.

How common is Parkinson's disease?

In the US, about 1 million people have PD, and as many as 10 million people have it worldwide, or approximately 3 out of every 1,000 individuals in industrialized countries. Older people experience PD more often; in fact, about 30 out of every 1,000 people older than the age of 80 have Parkinson's.

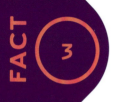

Approximately 30 out of every 1,000 people older than the age of 80 have Parkinson's.

Typical age at diagnosis

As people age, their chances of getting PD increases. Most cases of PD are diagnosed in people older than 50 years of age. The highest number of cases has been reported among people 85 to 89 years of age, although Parkinson's can still occur in people younger than age 50. If it is diagnosed before age 50, it is called **early-onset Parkinson's disease** (also known as young-onset PD). People who develop the disease at a young age are more likely to have a family history of Parkinson's.

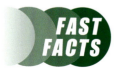

People with early-onset PD tend to have:
- More severe non-motor symptoms
- Slower progression of symptoms
- Better response to treatments
- Longer survival

People with early-onset PD are at a different point in their life when diagnosed. They may prioritize career and family considerations over health. It is important to work with a health care provider to address these concerns when creating a care plan. Because young-onset PD may run in families, genetic testing and counseling options for family planning may be considered.

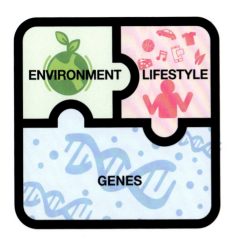
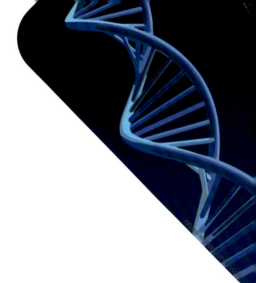

Are there factors that increase the risk for Parkinson's disease?

Several risk factors have been identified that may increase one's risk for Parkinson's. Generally, they are grouped within genetic, environmental, and lifestyle considerations. These factors may include:

• A family history of PD	• Exposure to pesticides
• >65 years of age	• Drinking well water
• History of head injury	• Male gender
• Working in agriculture (such as a farmer or fruit or vegetable picker)	• Caucasian race

The term **juvenile PD** is used for children and teenagers whose onset of PD occurs when they are younger than 20 years of age. In most cases, juvenile PD is due to genetic mutations.

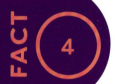

FACT 4

At least 15 genes have been identified for possible association with Parkinson's.

Risk factors (cont)

The link between some risk factors and PD is not fully understood. For example, researchers do not know why men are more likely to get PD. Risk factors can be difficult to pinpoint because of the time that passes between exposure and the onset of symptoms.

Some risk factors and how they interact with each other may not yet be fully understood. Based on what we know today, PD risk factors act as **triggers**, **facilitators**, and **aggravators**.

- Triggers are the spark that kicks things off. They can take place decades before symptoms develop. However, most people exposed to these triggers will never develop Parkinson's disease because they don't have a facilitator.
- Facilitators enable the trigger to cause further damage. If triggers are the spark, facilitators fan the flames.
- Aggravators, as the name implies, aggravate the disease process and enable it to cause further damage and spread through the brain.

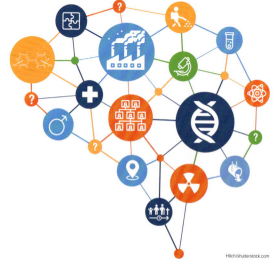

Hilch/shutterstock.com

50 FACTS & MORE

Every person diagnosed with PD may have experienced 1 or more triggers, facilitators, or aggravators in their lifetime, and may be exposed to additional facilitators and aggravators over time. Triggers, facilitators, and aggravators are different for each person, adding complexity in selecting participants for future clinical trials aiming to harness the promise of precision medicine.

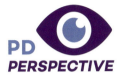

PD PERSPECTIVE

"I often say now I don't have any choice whether or not I have Parkinson's, but surrounding that non-choice is a million other choices that I can make."
–Michael J. Fox

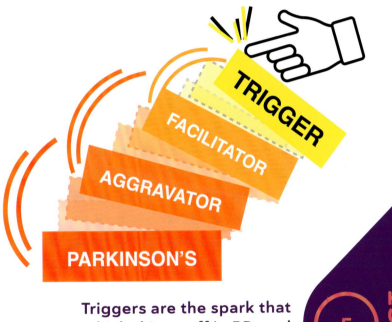

FACT 5

Triggers are the spark that kick things off in PD, and they often take place decades before symptoms develop. Each individual who develops Parkinson's is suspected to have a unique disease trigger.

Life With **PARKINSON'S**

How is Parkinson's disease diagnosed?

A diagnosis is based on a review of one's medical history, signs, symptoms, and observations. Symptoms often appear slowly and may not be immediately recognized as PD. Diagnosing Parkinson's is difficult, and there are no laboratory tests for it.

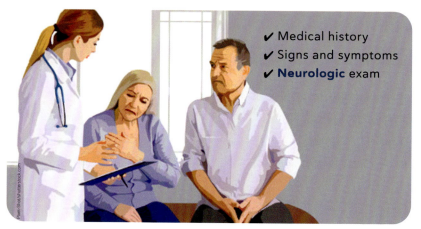

- ✔ Medical history
- ✔ Signs and symptoms
- ✔ **Neurologic** exam

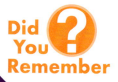

Did You Remember

Dopamine helps control movement. So, when the brain cannot make enough dopamine, symptoms related to difficulty with movement can appear.

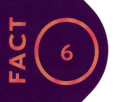

FACT 6

Diagnosing Parkinson's disease can be difficult.

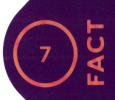

Men are nearly twice as likely as women to be diagnosed with Parkinson's.

FACT 7

What are motor symptoms?

Resting tremor, bradykinesia, and stiffness

Motor symptoms are usually the first and the most common signs of Parkinson's. **PD is diagnosed when at least 2 motor symptoms are present, 1 of which must be slow movements.**

> There are several types of motor symptoms. Some are more likely to occur in earlier stages than others. These make up the main symptoms that are used for diagnosis and include:
>
> - A resting tremor, which is an **involuntary rhythmic motion** that disappears with movement
> - Slow movements, called bradykinesia
> - Tightness and stiffness in the limbs, also called **rigidity**

COMMON MOTOR SYMPTOMS

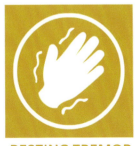

RESTING TREMOR

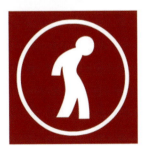

SLOWNESS IN MOVEMENT (BRADYKINESIA)

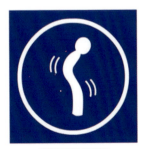

STIFFNESS RIGIDITY

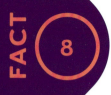

FACT 8

The number of PD cases is growing faster than for any other brain condition.

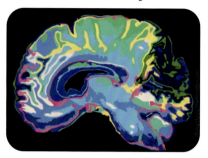

Other motor symptoms

In addition to the symptoms used for diagnosis, there are several other motor symptoms associated with PD. These symptoms are less common or may only develop much later in the course.

Additional Less Common Motor Symptoms in PD

- Problems with balance are called **postural instability**. People with postural instability have problems maintaining an upright posture when walking or standing. They may appear to lean slightly forward, which can lead to falls

- People with PD may have a walking pattern consisting of short steps that look like shuffling with limited arm swinging. In some cases, the stride may freeze, which means the person is unable to move forward. **Freezing** may look like the person is stuck in the middle of a step

- **Dystonia** is another motor symptom that may occur. Dystonia refers to uncontrolled muscle contractions in the legs, arms, neck, eyes, or trunk. The muscle movement can cause twisting or bending motions. This can be painful and affect the ability to do certain activities

50 FACTS & MORE

A resting tremor can occur in the jaw, chin, mouth, or tongue, as well as the arms and legs. Sometimes a **tremor** is felt but not seen, and this is called an **inner tremor**.

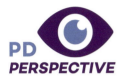

Then and Now, Life Is Still Good

"Imagine yourself then, imagine yourself now with Parkinson's. What are the differences? Life was good back then, and life is still good. The strength and resilience of friendships then were ever-present, and now this is even more important. The bonds in love before were strong but now even more crucial to augment survival."

Adapted with permission from Frank C. Church, *Imagine Yourself Then, Imagine Yourself Now With Parkinson's*

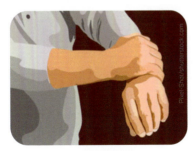

Tremor associated with PD usually starts on one side of the body. As the condition progresses, the tremor may spread to both sides.

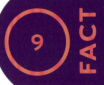

FACT 9

Further evaluation & diagnosis

Beyond motor symptoms, there are a few additional ways to support a PD diagnosis including:

- Improvement of symptoms with levodopa, the most important replacement of dopamine in the brain
- Existence of additional non-motor symptoms, such as loss of smell, **constipation**, depression, and/or **dream enactment behaviors**

Who can diagnose Parkinson's disease?

Primary care providers can diagnose PD based on symptoms; however, a doctor specializing in brain conditions, called a **neurologist**, can confirm the diagnosis. Neurologists with additional training in movement disorders are called **movement disorder specialists**. There are several conditions that can easily be confused for PD. A specialist can rule out these conditions and serve as a second opinion. People with PD who have severe symptoms may also see a movement disorder specialist for treatment of certain symptoms.

Parkinson's disease was first recognized by British surgeon Dr. James Parkinson.

*In 1817, British surgeon Dr. James Parkinson referred to the disease in his influential paper "The Essay on the **Shaking Palsy**."*

Artist's Rendition

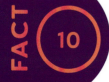

About 9 of 10 people with PD eventually lose their sense of smell. This is called anosmia.

Neurologists with specific training in movement disorders are called movement disorder specialists.

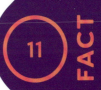

Role of imaging

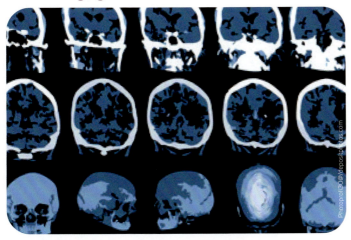

If a Parkinson's diagnosis remains unclear, an imaging test such as **DaTscan** or **magnetic resonance imaging (MRI)** may be used.

A DaTscan is a test involving a gamma camera that takes pictures of your brain to measure dopamine-containing **neurons** involved in controlling movement. A DaTscan result can be useful for determining whether a person has PD instead of **essential tremor** or **drug-induced parkinsonism**.

An MRI looks at the structure of the brain, and can help determine if specific regions of the brain are smaller than they should be, also known as **atrophy**. Brain structures in people diagnosed with PD are normal when evaluated by MRI.

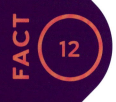

FACT 12

A change in handwriting, specifically handwriting that's gotten smaller over time or crowded, is called **micrographia**, and may be an early indicator of PD.

It is not in the stars to hold our destiny but in ourselves

It is not in the stars to hold our destiny but in ourselves
It is not in the stars to hold our destiny but in ourselves
It is not in the stars to hold our destiny but in ourself
It is not in the stars to hold our destiny but in ourselves

What are non-motor symptoms and complications?

Below is an introduction to many of the most common **non-motor PD symptoms**. In section 2, **these and other non-motor symptoms are discussed in greater detail along with "what to do about" them**. Although these are typical symptoms, they can vary greatly amongst individuals with PD in terms of their intensity and how they progress. Non-motor symptoms, sometimes called invisible symptoms, may appear years before movement (motor) symptoms. **As further discussed in section 2**, they may also be related to the deficiency of dopamine, or may happen for other reasons. Some people with Parkinson's may have several non-motor symptoms, whereas others may have few or none.

Cognitive symptoms

Cognitive symptoms in PD are non-motor impairments that may be an important cause of distress for people with Parkinson's including:

• Trouble finding words	• Confusion
• Poor decision making	• Problems with multitasking
• Changes in thinking	• Challenges completing everyday activities

Cognitive impairment typically appears over time and is more common with age. Early onset of cognitive difficulties may be a sign that PD is an incorrect diagnosis.

Psychiatric symptoms
Hallucinations/Psychosis, depression, and anxiety

Some people with PD also have psychiatric symptoms or mental health conditions. About 35% of people diagnosed with PD will experience depression. About 60% of people with PD will have anxiety. These symptoms can be present in the early stages of PD, and may even occur before PD is diagnosed. The severity of these symptoms differs among people. Depression and anxiety may get better with the same treatment used for motor symptoms or by directly addressing them with specific support that may include medicine.

Parkinson's disease psychosis

Some people with advanced PD may eventually come to **hallucinate** or have **delusions**. Hallucinations are when someone hears, feels, or smells something that is not real, whereas delusions are typically irrational beliefs that are not based on reality and resist any evidence to the contrary. Together, or separately, these behaviors are called Parkinson's disease psychosis. About 40% of people with PD eventually develop Parkinson's disease psychosis (PDP), which tends to occur late in the progression of Parkinson's.

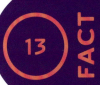

In addition to the well-known effects of boosting heart and lung function and slowing down cognitive decline, exercise can help improve gait, balance, walking ability, flexibility, and strength in people with Parkinson's.

Life With **PARKINSON'S**

Additional non-motor symptoms and complications

Extreme changes in behavior
People with PD may experience extreme changes in behavior such as **impulse control disorder (ICD)** and **pseudobulbar affect (PBA)**.

ICD includes gambling, excessive shopping, or making hasty or reckless choices. The most common strategy to deal with ICD is to slowly lower the dose of levodopa or dopamine agonist, and adjust the doses of other medicines. Another possible consideration may be to stop using a dopamine agonist completely, in favor of another choice of medicine.

Some people with PD may also laugh or cry uncontrollably for no reason. They may laugh without mirth or cry without sadness. This is called the pseudobulbar affect.

Many non-motor symptoms of PD are treatable. Write down these "invisible symptoms" if and when they present and then discuss them with your doctors to seek treatment.

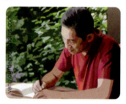

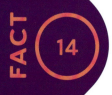

Freezing of gait can last from just a few to up to 30 seconds for most of those affected with this motor problem. In rare cases, the person may not be able to return to forward motion for several minutes.

Neurogenic orthostatic hypotension (NOH) is experienced by 50% of people with PD.

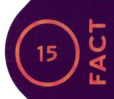

FACT 15

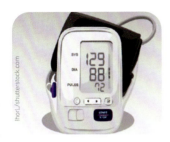

Falls related to Parkinson's disease

People with Parkinson's may be at higher risk for injury due to falling. The most common cause of falls in people with PD is freezing of gait, which is the inability to lift one's feet off the ground when walking, often while turning or changing directions or when attempting to do so. As freezing brings the body to a sudden halt, forward falls can occur. A contributing problem is related to the development of a **stooped** posture, which adds to the likelihood that any freezing episode will cause this type of fall.

There are several additional contributing factors discussed here that also may increase the possibility of falls in people with PD, such as **neurogenic orthostatic hypotension (NOH)** and impaired **postural reflexes**.

Neurogenic orthostatic hypotension

Neurogenic orthostatic hypotension in PD is common and refers to a drop in blood pressure that occurs when standing up. It can also happen when going from lying down to sitting up. This can cause lightheadedness and dizziness and lead to a fall with or without fainting.

Postural reflexes

Another reason for falls related to PD is impairment in postural reflexes. Postural reflexes keep the body upright and aligned. PD lowers one's ability to remain upright when exposed to external forces, such as bumping against something or someone, leading to falls forward or to the side.

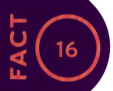

It is more common for people with Parkinson's to have problems staying asleep than falling asleep.

Additional non-motor symptoms and complications (cont)

Sleep problems

It is common to have trouble sleeping with PD. You may have a hard time falling asleep, staying asleep, or both. **This is called insomnia.** People with Parkinson's may also experience daytime sleepiness from PD-related causes such as getting up frequently during the night to go to the bathroom (see bladder issues, page 33).

People with PD-related motor symptoms may have trouble adjusting sleeping positions to get comfortable in bed. Others may experience hallucinations when trying to fall asleep. Sometimes, due to insomnia or other causes, people with PD may also experience **excessive daytime sleepiness (EDS)**.

Because both depression and anxiety can contribute to insomnia, these conditions may also lead to sleep problems in people with Parkinson's. Insomnia, daytime sleepiness, depression, and anxiety are discussed in greater detail in section 2.

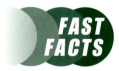

The same type of stiffness and slowness that can impact walking and other activities in people with PD can appear as reduced facial expression, also called hypomimia or facial masking. When the muscles of the face are stiff or take longer to move, it can be difficult to smile, raise eyebrows, or express feelings using facial muscles, making it hard for others to interpret mood and intentions.

Constipation and bladder issues

Constipation is common for those with Parkinson's, and it can range from a mild nuisance that causes temporary discomfort to a more chronic problem that significantly affects quality of life. For some, constipation can impact the effectiveness of medicines for PD. Constipation can occur at any time during the course of Parkinson's, sometimes even decades before the disease is diagnosed. Constipation can be a side effect of medicines taken for PD as well.

For people with Parkinson's, bladder issues are often due to changes in dopamine levels affecting the bladder's muscles and nerves, which are critical to how it functions. You may also have issues with urinating. This may be an increase in urgency or frequency. Urgency is a feeling of needing to urinate right away. Frequency is the need to go often. When these issues occur more often during the night, it is referred to as **nocturia**.

Speech, voice, and swallowing

PD can affect the use of many of the muscles used for speech, chewing, and swallowing. They may move more slowly due to bradykinesia and cause speech changes over time. PD may also impact how speech is controlled in the brain.

Some people with advanced PD, especially those with swallowing problems, may experience excessive drooling, called **sialorrhea**, because they swallow less often and saliva can build up.

Parkinson's can cause a reduction in **autonomic functions**, including swallowing. Difficulty with swallowing is called **dysphagia**.

Did you know? Although tremors are probably the most well-known signs of Parkinson's, around 20% to 25% of people with Parkinson's *never* actually develop them.

Additional non-motor symptoms and complications (cont)

Pain

Between 40% and 80% of people with Parkinson's experience pain at some point. This may or may not be directly due to their disease. There are 5 types of pain that may be caused or intensified by PD.

Musculoskeletal pain: This is muscle, bone, or joint pain caused by many non-PD conditions such as arthritis. Stiff muscles or poor posture caused by PD may worsen musculoskeletal pain caused by other conditions.

Dystonia pain: This is pain due to an abnormal posture of a foot, hand, or neck as part of the motor abnormalities of PD or due to fluctuations with the medicines used in the treatment of PD and its symptoms.

Nerve pain: This pain can be a burning or shooting feeling due to damage in the small nerves in the feet and/or can be related to pressure exerted on a nerve exiting the spinal cord. Poor posture and stiff muscles in PD can make nerve pain worse.

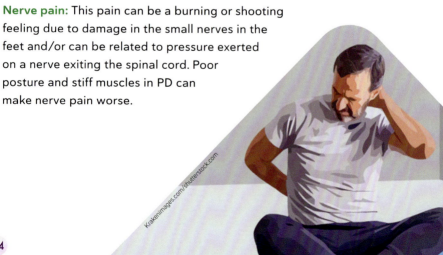

Central pain: This can be described as a deep pain, but the feeling varies from person to person. It may feel like an aching, burning, or stabbing sensation and is also the rarest pain syndrome experienced by people with PD.

Depression and pain: People with PD and depression report greater pain severity and more disability related to pain, compared with people with PD without depression. Depression must be considered as a contributing factor in assessing pain in people with PD.

As discussed in section 2, it is important to talk to your health care provider if you have pain. They can help determine the cause so that you can get proper treatment.

Melanoma

People with PD have a higher risk of developing melanoma, a type of skin cancer. Decreased exposure to the sun can help prevent melanoma. Consider visiting a dermatologist, a doctor who treats skin disorders, once a year for a skin evaluation. Melanoma is easier to treat if it is detected early.

You can reduce sun exposure by wearing protective clothing. Use a waterproof sunscreen that is at least SPF 30 for any exposed skin.

Every 9 minutes, someone in the US is diagnosed with PD.

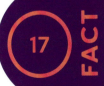

Life With **PARKINSON'S**

What is the goal of treating Parkinson's disease?

The need to individualize treatment

The goal of PD treatment is to improve the motor and non-motor symptoms discussed previously in this section. Understanding the causes and the treatment approaches available for addressing these symptoms is discussed in section 2. As PD progresses, it may become harder to perform normal activities, such as getting dressed, eating, or keeping a job. Treatment with medicines can help you meet personal functional expectations of daily living while improving your overall quality of life. Treatment will be based on each person's symptoms and individual circumstances. Different treatment options may be preferred depending on which symptoms are most troublesome.

Your doctor will consider many factors when deciding on the best treatment for your PD, including:

• Your age	• Other conditions you may have
• The severity of your PD	• Your preferences for treatment

People with PD often experience mood changes and, therefore may withdraw from seeking help. Talking about such symptoms with a health care provider helps create a greater overall sense of "control." This then enables providers to better understand how PD is having an impact and suggest solutions.

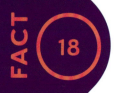

Studies show that high-intensity exercise, such as running on a treadmill for 30 minutes 3 times a week, can considerably delay the progression of Parkinson's, which can have an enormous impact over time.

People with PD are experiencing healthier and longer life spans. They are living longer and better.

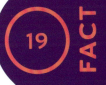

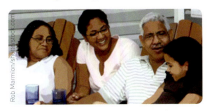

Lifestyle strategies

In general, and especially for those with Parkinson's, regular exercise combined with a healthy diet are important for overall health. If you have PD, getting enough of the right kind of exercise daily is critical, as it can improve strength, endurance, mobility, flexibility, balance, walking ability, and sleep. These are all critical factors contributing to one's quality of life, especially for people with Parkinson's.

Diet

People with PD should eat a healthy diet low in carbohydrates but normal in fat and cholesterol (the brain is filled with cholesterol; a good amount of it is important). Olive oil, eggs, nuts, and fish are excellent sources of fat. Try to eat plenty of fruits and vegetables, particularly those that are colorful or dark in color because they are high in **antioxidants.** Foods that are high in fiber (whole grains, brown rice, and beans) can also help with digestion. Milk, dairy products, and fish are good sources of vitamin D, which helps to keep bones healthy.

We have all grown up with the idea of the importance of limiting the intake of salt to prevent high blood pressure. For those with PD, however, there is more of a tendency for low blood pressure. In these circumstances, high water and salt intake may be recommended by a health care provider.

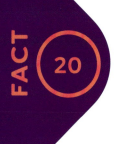

FACT 20

Sports and exercise regimens, such as walking, biking, yoga, and tai chi, have been shown to improve balance, motor control, and strength in people with PD. Physical and occupational therapy can also aid in improving gait, flexibility, and speech.

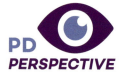

PD PERSPECTIVE

"With Parkinson's, exercise is better than taking a bottle of pills. If you don't do anything, you'll just stagnate."
–Brian Lambert

Exercise

Regular exercise is safe and recommended for those with PD due to its many benefits. A well-rounded exercise program should include activities for endurance, strength, flexibility, and balance. Exercise plans and goals may be individualized by a health care professional, and can be modified as symptoms change. **The Davis Phinney Foundation for Parkinson's** provides a wide range of workouts designed specifically for people with Parkinson's disease that can be modified to match one's fitness level (davisphinneyfoundation.org/parkinsons-exercise-essentials-video).

Dental care

Symptoms of PD can make brushing and flossing teeth difficult; therefore, people with Parkinson's may experience dental issues. Some examples include cracking or wearing down of teeth and changes in how dentures fit. A lack of saliva may occur in some people with PD, as a result of some medicines, and can make them more prone to cavities.

Symptoms of PD can interfere with regular dental care. Suggestions that can make dental appointments run as smoothly as possible include:

• Inform the dentist about your PD symptoms before your appointment	• Provide the dentist with an updated list of current medicines
• Schedule appointments at times of the day when symptoms are less likely to be problematic	• Try to avoid delaying major dental work

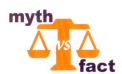

MYTH: *"Your doctor can predict your specific Parkinson's progression and trajectory."*

FACT: Parkinson's is unique for each person. Even a PD expert has no way of knowing what the future holds for each individual.

If you are exercising with moderate intensity, you should be able to talk, but not sing. If you are only able to get a few words out when talking, you are exercising vigorously.

Keywords & Concepts Introduced in Section 2*

- ✔ Acetylcholine (ACh)
- ✔ Adenosine A_{2a} antagonists
- ✔ Adherence
- ✔ Amantadine
- ✔ Amino acid
- ✔ Anticholinergic
- ✔ Apomorphine
- ✔ Blood-brain barrier
- ✔ Carbidopa
- ✔ Center of Excellence Network
- ✔ Central Nervous System (CNS)
- ✔ Cognitive function
- ✔ COMT Inhibitors
- ✔ Deep brain stimulation (DBS)
- ✔ Device-aided Parkinson therapies
- ✔ Diphasic dyskinesia
- ✔ Dopamine agonists (DAs)
- ✔ Dopamine receptor
- ✔ Droxidopa
- ✔ Dyskinesia
- ✔ Enlarged prostate
- ✔ Entacapone
- ✔ Enzymes
- ✔ Executive function
- ✔ Extended-release (ER)
- ✔ Fludrocortisone
- ✔ Globus pallidus
- ✔ Infusion
- ✔ Istradefylline
- ✔ Levodopa/carbidopa intestinal gel (LCIG) infusion
- ✔ Levodopa (L-dopa)
- ✔ MAO-B Inhibitors
- ✔ Midodrine
- ✔ Molecules
- ✔ Motor fluctuations
- ✔ Neuropsychologist
- ✔ Occupational therapist
- ✔ "Off" episodes
- ✔ "On" episodes
- ✔ Opicapone
- ✔ Overstimulation
- ✔ Pallidotomy
- ✔ Parkinson's Foundation
- ✔ Peak-dose dyskinesia
- ✔ Peak level
- ✔ Personal health literacy
- ✔ Pramipexole
- ✔ Primer
- ✔ Ropinirole
- ✔ Rotigotine
- ✔ Serotonin
- ✔ Side effects
- ✔ Signals
- ✔ Signal transmission
- ✔ Sleep-wake cycle
- ✔ Social worker
- ✔ Speech-language therapist
- ✔ Synapse
- ✔ Team-based approach
- ✔ Titration
- ✔ Tolcapone
- ✔ Tyrosine
- ✔ Urinary tract infection
- ✔ Urologist
- ✔ Vivid dreams
- ✔ "Wearing-off" effect

*Terms listed here are addressed in this section and can be found with their definitions in the Glossary (page 196).

SECTION 2: PARKINSON'S DISEASE & TREATMENTS

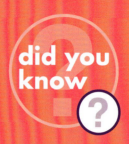

Personal health literacy is the degree to which individuals have the ability to find, understand, and use information and services to inform their health-related decisions and decide actions for themselves and others. Low health literacy is associated with poorer outcomes for people with Parkinson's as well as an increased burden for their support team members and family.

PARKINSON'S DISEASE & TREATMENTS

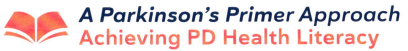

A Parkinson's Primer Approach
Achieving PD Health Literacy

| Understanding the Mechanics of Parkinson's Disease | Understanding Treatment Approaches for Motor Symptoms With Medicine | Understanding Treatment Approaches for Motor Symptoms (Device & Surgery) | Overview of Non-Motor Symptoms & Approaches |

Parkinson's disease (PD) is a complex and multifaceted illness—and it can be intimidating. An analogy might be our modern cars, which are such complicated machines that most of us must turn to a mechanic whenever something is wrong, rather than trying to understand and attempt a fix ourselves. Similarly, people with PD turn to a doctor when they experience symptoms. However, unlike a vehicle that stays in the garage when not in use, *you are always in your body*, and so you and your family will naturally want to understand more about the *Mechanics of PD* including the "how and why's" of symptoms. Knowing more about how Parkinson's operates, and how treatments aim to help with PD symptoms (both motor and non-motor) empowers people with Parkinson's, their caregivers, and the family support network.

Why a primer approach? A primer is a traditional, time-proven way to teach complex subjects using simple terms and examples, clear writing, and imagery. The goal is to educate effectively without overwhelming. Overall, **The PD Companion** is designed to do just that, **and section 2 specifically,** thereby increasing PD-related health literacy for the interested reader. Some readers may find the level of detail to follow to be "just right," whereas others may wish to delve even more deeply into specific topics by consulting additional sources.

Understanding the underlying causes of your motor and non-motor PD symptoms—and how they can be addressed with various treatments—can help you manage your own unique circumstances. Because PD is a progressive disease, symptom changes over time may be related to aging, changes in how your body responds to medicines, or changes in how your brain is working. It is important that you maintain regular contact with your **health care team** to discuss any change in symptoms or new symptoms that you experience. These changes may suggest that it is time to update your treatment plan and/or adjust your medicines to support your functional expectations of daily living and overall quality of life.

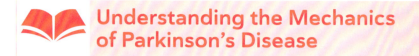

Understanding the Mechanics of Parkinson's Disease

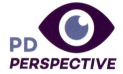

PD PERSPECTIVE

"You've survived 100% of everything in your life so far, so there's a pretty good chance that you'll survive whatever is next."
—Timber Hawkeye

How do neurons work to make muscles move?

Neurons are the fundamental units of the brain and nervous system. These cells are responsible for sending motor (movement) **signals** to our muscles, and for transforming and relaying signals at every step in between.

To send and receive these signals, nerve cells rely on 2 forms of **signal transmission**—electrical and chemical.

Neurons send signals from one end of a cell to the other as electric impulses. When the impulse reaches the far end of the nerve cell, a neurotransmitter (a chemical) is released into the space between 2 nerve cells, also known as the **synapse** (Figure 1). In the substantia nigra, *dopamine is the neurotransmitter* that sends signals from one nerve cell to the next, to control movement. **As described in section 1, the major cause of motor symptoms in PD is the loss of dopamine in the substantia nigra.**

PARKINSON'S DISEASE & TREATMENTS

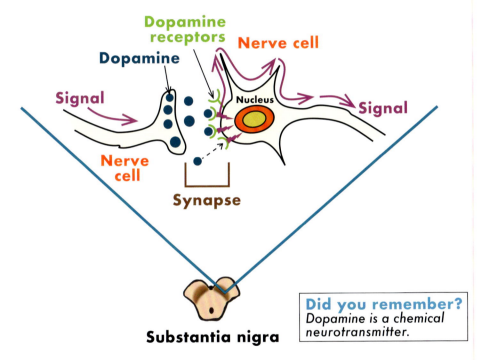

Figure 1 Signal Transmissions (electrical impulses) Moving *ALONG* 2 Nerve Cells (called neurons) and *BETWEEN* Cells Via Chemical Transmission (dopamine).

Did you remember?
Dopamine is a chemical neurotransmitter.

Outside the substantia nigra, neurons use different types of neurotransmitters to send signals from one neuron to the next, such as **acetylcholine (ACh)** which is discussed further on page 71.

Life With **PARKINSON'S**

Mechanics of PD

Dopamine released into the synapse moves across the synapse and finds (binds to) a **dopamine receptor** on the next neuron, much like a thrown baseball ends up in the pocket of a friend's baseball glove during a game of catch.

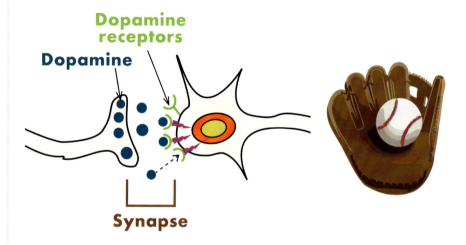

The dopamine receptor is very specific, it only "catches" dopamine, **or a limited number of molecules that "look like" dopamine** (which will be important to remember when we discuss treatment). When dopamine is "caught" by this receptor, a new electric impulse is generated in the next neuron (nerve cell), **and the "signal" continues to be transmitted along the second neuron**. This process of electrical-chemical-electrical signal transmission is repeated at each synapse along the chain of neurons that connects the brain, spine, and nerves to individual muscles, which transforms signals from the brain into actual "movement" in the body.

PARKINSON'S DISEASE & TREATMENTS

How do neurons in the substantia nigra get their dopamine?

The brain is protected by a **blood-brain barrier (BBB)** that controls what does or doesn't enter the brain from the bloodstream. For example, the BBB allows **tyrosine**, an **amino acid** that neurons use to *make* dopamine (see below), to move from the blood into the brain, but the BBB does not allow fully formed dopamine to move from blood to the brain (Figure 2).

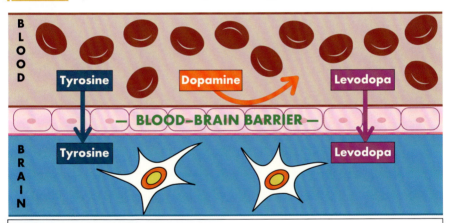

Figure 2 Tyrosine and Levodopa Crossing the Blood–Brain Barrier.

Did you remember?
Fully formed dopamine cannot pass through the blood–brain barrier; however, both naturally occurring tyrosine (amino acid) and levodopa can (levodopa is an important medicine introduced on page 53). Each are then used to make dopamine.

An amino acid is a basic substance in your body that serves as a building block for proteins. Nerve cells in the brain (substantia nigra) use an amino acid called tyrosine to make dopamine.

Life With **PARKINSON'S**

Mechanics of PD

Since dopamine is not delivered "whole" to the brain, how is it actually made?

Healthy neurons in the substantia nigra make the dopamine they need from the amino acid tyrosine which

- Is normally available in blood,
- Can cross the blood-brain barrier, and
- Can be taken into neurons.

Tyrosine is taken inside neurons and is first converted to **L-dopa**, then into dopamine. After this process, newly made dopamine is stored near the end of the neuron, ready to be released into the synapse when an electrical impulse (signal) arrives. Once released into the synapse, dopamine moves across the open space to the next neuron, where it is caught by the dopamine receptor (Figure 3).

Figure 3 Important Steps for Making New Dopamine, Storage, and Release by Nerve Cells (Neurons).

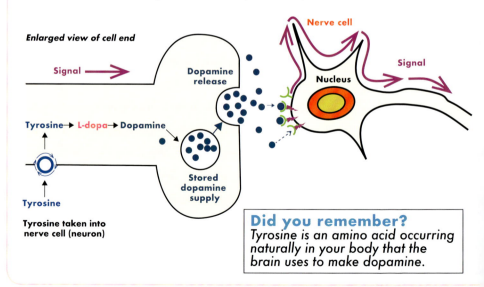

Did you remember?
Tyrosine is an amino acid occurring naturally in your body that the brain uses to make dopamine.

PARKINSON'S DISEASE & TREATMENTS

Some dopamine actually needs to be eliminated!

After all the discussion on the importance of dopamine in **PD**, it may be hard to believe that some dopamine released into the synapse eventually **needs to be eliminated** (Figure 4). This process must occur in order to prevent a build up of excess dopamine, as **too much** dopamine can also cause movement disorders known as **dyskinesia** (page 62).

Dopamine is eliminated by 2 special **enzymes**: **monoamine oxidase type b (MAO-B)** and/or **catechol-O-methyltransferase (COMT)**. Each of these enzymes breaks down dopamine into fragments that can no longer interact with dopamine receptors. **Medicine is available that can block each of these enzymes, thereby helping to preserve dopamine levels for people with PD** (page 66).

Figure 4 Dopamine Supply in the Brain Is a Balance Between New Dopamine Production and Dopamine Breakdown.

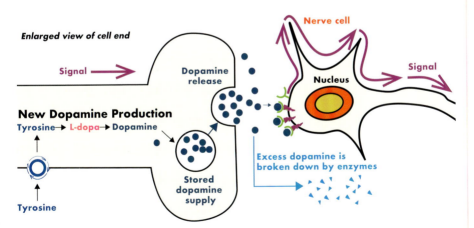

Did you remember?
Too much dopamine in the brain can cause dyskinesia.

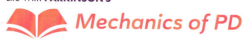

Mechanics of PD

Balancing dopamine production & elimination

There is normally a delicate, fine-tuned balancing act between dopamine production and elimination that controls the amount of dopamine available for use by the neuron. **This balancing act is regulated with no difficulty in people who do not have PD** (Figure 5).

Figure 5 The Balance Between New Dopamine and Dopamine Breakdown Regulates Amount of Dopamine Available For Communication Between Nerve Cells.

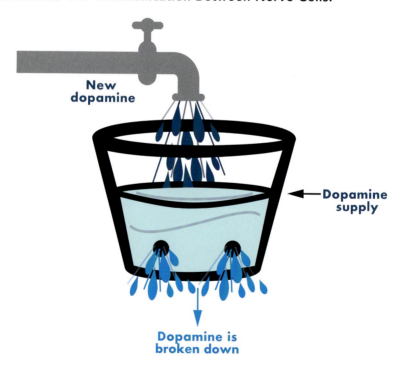

PARKINSON'S DISEASE & TREATMENTS

For people with PD, however, this balancing act needs to be adjusted to help maintain adequate supplies of dopamine (Figure 6). These adjustments can be made with medicines that increase the overall supply of dopamine available, or those that can slow the elimination process of dopamine in the brain (Figures 7, 8, 11, and 12).

Figure 6 Less New Dopamine Leads to Low Dopamine Supply.

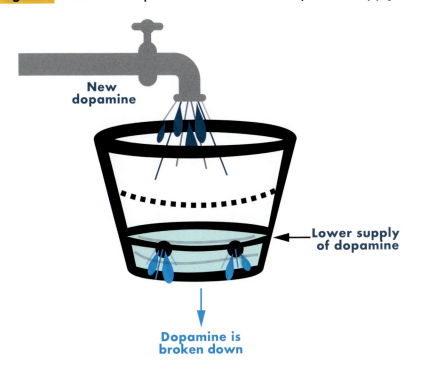

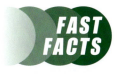 Dopamine is broken down (eliminated) by 2 special enzymes: MAO-B and COMT (page 66).

Understanding Treatment Approaches for Motor Symptoms With Medicine

There are 3 approaches to the treatment of PD motor symptoms with medicines to correct (treat) low dopamine levels in the substantia nigra of people with Parkinson's:

1	By increasing the amount of actual dopamine available for use (page 53)
2	By providing the brain with an accepted substitute medicine to take the place of the missing dopamine (page 64)
3	By slowing the natural dopamine elimination (break down) process (page 66)

did you know?

Having a medical care team is strongly recommended by the Parkinson's Foundation. With a **team-based approach**, different experts work with you on an as-needed basis to address your full range of symptoms. More information on this approach can be found on the **Parkinson's Foundation** website, including information about their "**Center of Excellence Network**," which is widely recognized as among the best-in-class treatment centers for Parkinson's. Find out more @parkinson.org.

PARKINSON'S DISEASE & TREATMENTS

Q If the lack of dopamine causes motor symptoms in people with Parkinson's, are there ways to increase the amount of dopamine available?

A To treat low dopamine levels in people with PD, medicine is available (levodopa also called L-dopa) that can increase dopamine levels. In fact, levodopa is considered the most important medicine designed to treat the lack of dopamine and the related motor symptoms in PD.

1 Treating low dopamine levels in people with Parkinson's

Levodopa (L-dopa)

As discussed in section 1, people with PD are not able to maintain enough dopamine in the substantia nigra. This low dopamine level causes the disruption of the normal control of nerve function and body movement. To treat the low dopamine levels in people with PD, medicine is available (levodopa, also called L-dopa) that can increase dopamine levels. When taken by mouth, levodopa is absorbed by the intestine and travels through the bloodstream to the brain. Just like tyrosine (page 47), levodopa can also cross the blood-brain barrier and be taken into neurons. In the neurons, levodopa is converted into dopamine, thereby replacing the missing dopamine in people with Parkinson's and restoring their motor function (Figures 7 and 8).

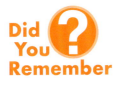

Levodopa is the cornerstone of PD treatment. It helps increase dopamine levels in your brain and ease motor symptoms, which are largely caused by having too little dopamine (page 3).

Life With **PARKINSON'S**

Motor Symptoms & Medicines

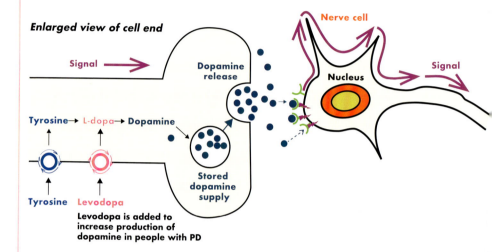

Figure 7 Adding Levodopa Can Increase Available Supply of Dopamine in Individuals With Parkinson's Disease.

Levodopa is added to increase production of dopamine in people with PD

Did you remember?
BOTH naturally occurring tyrosine and levodopa (medicine) can enter nerve cells (neurons) to make dopamine.

Levodopa therapy is typically started as soon as motor symptoms become bothersome. The amount of levodopa needed varies from person to person. To minimize the possibility of **side effects**, it is best to have your body get used to taking levodopa slowly, so it is normally taken in smaller amounts that can be increased gradually over time to eventually achieve control of PD motor symptoms. This slow increase of medicine over time is called **titration**. Titration may alleviate some side effects that may normally occur at the start of treatment with levodopa.

50 FACTS & MORE

PARKINSON'S DISEASE & TREATMENTS

Figure 8 Taking Levodopa Can Increase Dopamine Levels In Parkinson's Disease.

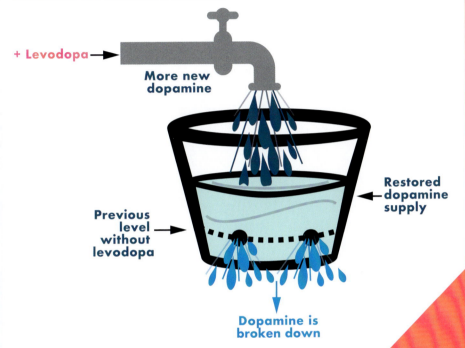

Levodopa is the most effective medicine for treating the motor symptoms of PD. Levodopa and L-dopa mean the same thing. L-dopa is an abbreviation of Levodopa.

FACT 22

Life With **PARKINSON'S**

Motor Symptoms & Medicines

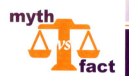

MYTH: *"Levodopa stops working after 5 years."* This is a pervasive PD treatment myth.

FACT: Levodopa will always work for as long as the person lives. Levodopa does not treat all the symptoms of PD, but it dramatically helps the most disabling motor symptoms.

Carbidopa

It is important to understand that enzymes, outside of the brain, can convert levodopa to other chemicals, thereby reducing the amount of levodopa that reaches the brain. **To prevent this "outside the brain" use of levodopa, carbidopa is always given with the levodopa. Carbidopa prevents the body from transforming levodopa before it reaches the brain.** As a result, taking carbidopa means that less overall levodopa medicine is needed. Carbidopa protects **BOTH** the natural levodopa in your body **AND** the medicine form of it. This increases overall dopamine availability in the brain, which also helps reduce **side effects**.

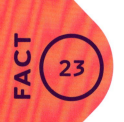

FACT 23 — Carbidopa is always given with levodopa.

50 FACTS & MORE

PARKINSON'S DISEASE & TREATMENTS

Levodopa is the best medicine for treating PD at any age. However, other medicines may also be used in young people with PD, or in people with milder symptoms. Your doctor will work with you to weigh the risks and benefits of each treatment to decide which options can best help you manage your functional expectations of daily living.

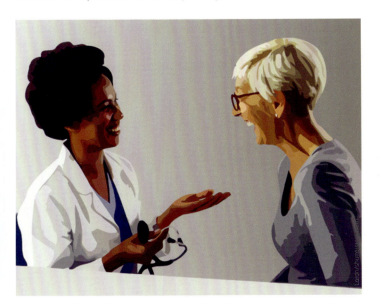

Carbidopa/levodopa comes in several different forms: as a tablet, a capsule, an orally disintegrating tablet, and a liquid suspension that can be directly infused into the intestine. You can talk with your health care provider about which may be best for your goals.

FACT 24

Life With **PARKINSON'S**

Motor Symptoms & Medicines

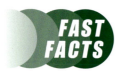 Carbidopa also protects your body's naturally occurring levodopa to provide even more for your brain.

Carbidopa
+
Levodopa from medicine
+
Body's natural levodopa

=

More levodopa going to just the brain

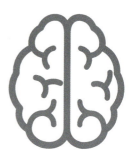

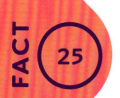 Carbidopa/levodopa only works for a few hours at a time, so they usually need to be taken several times a day.

PARKINSON'S DISEASE & TREATMENTS

Motor fluctuations

After a dose of levodopa is taken by mouth, the level of levodopa in the bloodstream increases to a maximum level called a **peak level**. From this peak, levels slowly decline over time as levodopa is naturally eliminated from the body. Because of this pattern of peaks followed by declining levels, people taking levodopa will experience what are known as **"on" episodes**—times when levodopa levels are sufficient for adequate symptom control—and **"off" episodes** when there is not enough levodopa to control the symptoms in the same way. This pattern of "on" and "off" episodes is known as motor fluctuations (Figure 9).

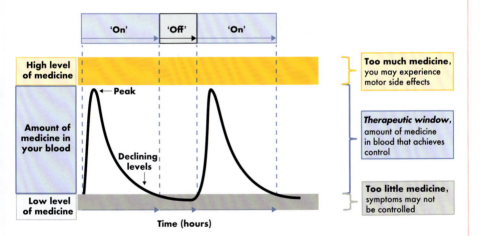

Figure 9 Amount (Concentration) of Medicine in Blood Over Time, After Taking Each Dose of Levodopa by Mouth.

You can contact the creators of *The PD Companion* directly with comments, suggestions, and ideas for future updates by emailing *Info@50Facts.com*.

Life With **PARKINSON'S**

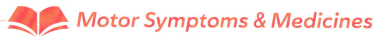
Motor Symptoms & Medicines

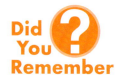

Too much dopamine can also cause movement disorders known as dyskinesia.

"Off" episodes

"Off" episode motor symptoms include tremor, stiffness, and difficulty with movement. Non-motor symptoms can include anxiety, fatigue, difficulty thinking, restlessness, or sweating. "Off" episode symptoms that occur at night can disrupt sleep. For some, "off" episode symptoms can appear suddenly and be disruptive.

Some people with PD may be reluctant to discuss "off" episode symptoms with a health care provider because they wrongly believe that the events are not avoidable, or because they are difficult to describe, or that the presence of these episodes may suggest that their Parkinson's is progressing. As it turns out, health care providers have several strategies that can minimize "off" episodes, so it's important to communicate about them with your doctor.

When "off" episodes become bothersome, interrupt your day, or interfere with your ability to work, your doctor may consider:

- Increasing how often you take levodopa, or switching you to a longer acting or **extended-release (ER)** version of levodopa.
- Giving you an additional (new types) medicine (discussed below) to make your "on" episode last longer each day.

"Wearing-off" effect refers to the tendency, after long-term levodopa treatment, for each dose of the medicine to become less effective before the next dose is due.

50 FACTS & MORE

PARKINSON'S DISEASE & TREATMENTS

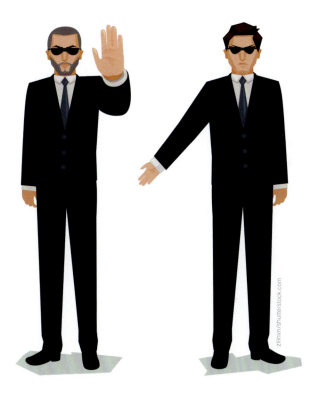

Levodopa needs to be taken with carbidopa or it will be used by the body in other locations before making it to the brain. Carbidopa is like a "bodyguard" for levodopa, to make sure it gets to where its supposed to, which makes sense because it's a "VIM"–Very Important Medicine– for those with Parkinson's.

FACT 26

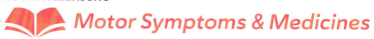

Motor Symptoms & Medicines

Overstimulation

Because the activity of substantia nigra in people with Parkinson's continues to slow over time, there is an increased need for levodopa as PD progresses.

If greater amounts of levodopa are needed to maintain good motor control, some overstimulation may occur, resulting in something called **peak-dose dyskinesia**. On page 49, the brain's balancing act with dopamine was described; overstimulation is caused by too much dopamine being present for a brief episode of time "at the peak." Symptoms of such overstimulation include experiencing uncontrollable "wiggly" or dance-like movements in the body, often in the trunk, neck, and arms. Peak-dose dyskinesia usually happens around 60 to 90 minutes after taking this larger amount of levodopa medicine. Another type of dyskinesia people with PD may experience is **diphasic dyskinesia**. This type of dyskinesia tends to affect the pelvis and legs, and **occurs around the time the medicine levels in the blood are declining, closer to the time the next dose of levodopa is due, or when the effect of the next dose has not yet kicked in fully (that is, when the dose of levodopa is working suboptimally).**

An inhaled form of levodopa is FDA-approved for rapid treatment of "off" episodes in people with Parkinson's who are taking regular levodopa therapy. Inhaled levodopa should not be substituted for your regular levodopa therapy, and may not be appropriate for those with chronic lung diseases such as asthma or chronic obstructive pulmonary disease.

50 FACTS & MORE

PARKINSON'S DISEASE & TREATMENTS

did you know?

Levodopa has been shown to improve the quality of life in people with PD.

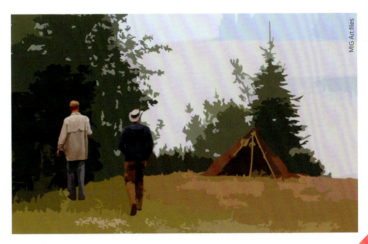

It is critical to take your doses of levodopa exactly on time, every time. Even so, "off" episodes can be expected when levodopa levels in your blood fall below the therapeutic range, especially in the morning before the first daily dose has taken effect. A medicine reminder can help you stay on schedule with your medicines, which is called **adherence**.

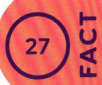

FACT 27

Life With **PARKINSON'S**

Motor Symptoms & Medicines

2 Providing the brain with an accepted substitute medicine to take the place of the lost dopamine

 If the lack of dopamine causes motor symptoms in people with Parkinson's, are there ways to provide the brain with an accepted substitute medicine to take the place of the lost dopamine?

Dopamine agonists (DA) are replacement medicines that can also cross the blood-brain barrier (page 47) and directly activate the same receptors that dopamine does (Figure 10).

Dopamine Agonists

DAs, including **apomorphine**, **pramipexole**, **ropinirole**, and **rotigotine**, are a type of medicine that can activate the brain's dopamine receptors, resulting in the same signal that dopamine produces when it is caught by the receptor. Unlike levodopa, DAs do not need to be converted into dopamine first. DAs do not work in the same exact way, or as effectively, as levodopa. Additionally, DAs do not specifically require carbidopa to ensure delivery to the brain like levodopa. DAs can be used to treat early, milder symptoms of PD. They can also be used in combination with carbidopa/levodopa to make the "on" episodes last longer. Apomorphine is a short-acting DA used in PD to treat "off" episodes that may not be sufficiently controlled by increasing the frequency or amount of levodopa taken (page 59).

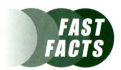 **Dopamine agonists are useful in treating motor symptoms because they can overcome or delay dyskinesia.**

PARKINSON'S DISEASE & TREATMENTS

Figure 10 Dopamine Agonists Can Substitute for Dopamine and Increase Supply in People With Parkinson's Disease.

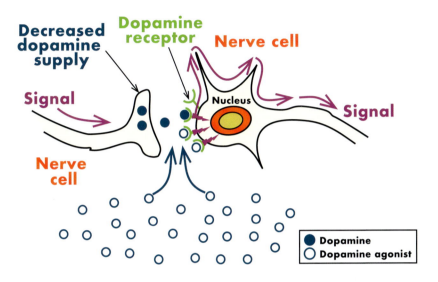

Dopamine agonists can cross the blood-brain barrier but do not specifically require carbidopa to ensure delivery to the brain like levodopa.

FACT 28

Life With **PARKINSON'S**

Motor Symptoms & Medicines

3 Slowing the dopamine elimination (breakdown) process

Two types of "breakdown" inhibitors are available for people with PD: MAO-B inhibitors and COMT inhibitors.

MAO-B inhibitors

MAO-B is an enzyme that breaks down neurotransmitters, including dopamine (Figure 4).

Medicines including **safinamide**, **selegiline**, and **rasagiline** "stop" or inhibit the activity of the MAO-B enzyme and are called ***MAO-B inhibitors***. They help maintain dopamine in the brain because they prevent MAO-B from breaking down dopamine (Figure 11). Like DAs, MAO-B inhibitors can help improve motor symptom control. They may be used alone by people with mild PD, or they may be combined with other medicines specifically to treat "off" episodes, by increasing the length of "on" episodes.

Figure 11 MAO-B Inhibitors Help Maintain Dopamine Supply.

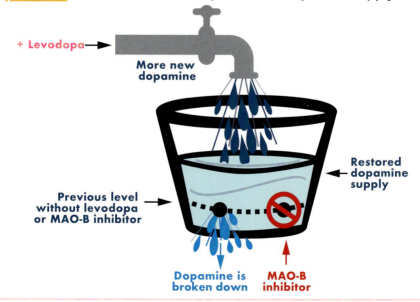

PARKINSON'S DISEASE & TREATMENTS

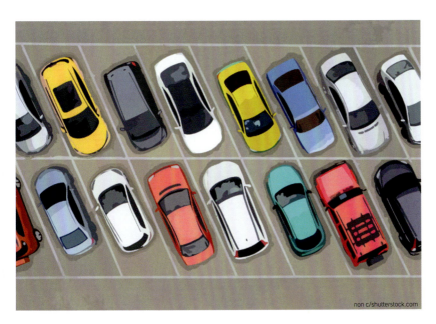

The Parking Lot Analogy. For people with PD, medicine that slows the breakdown of dopamine in the brain helps maintain dopamine levels. To better understand how this works, think about how a parking lot works outside a busy restaurant. Normally, people tip the attendant to get their car out of the lot as fast as possible, right? But what if everyone paid that same attendant to bring their car out *slower*? **What would happen to the lot? Of course it would stay fuller longer.**

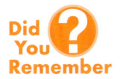

Adjustments to the brain's dopamine balancing act can be made with medicines that either slow the elimination process of dopamine in the brain, or increase the overall supply of dopamine (Figures 11 and 12).

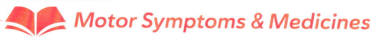

Motor Symptoms & Medicines

COMT inhibitors

COMT is an enzyme that breaks down neurotransmitters, including dopamine (Figure 4). Medicines that "stop" or *inhibit* the activity of the COMT enzyme are called *COMT inhibitors*. FDA-approved COMT inhibitors include **entacapone**, **tolcapone**, and **opicapone**. The way COMT inhibitors work is different from MAO-B inhibitors, but the benefit to dopamine supply in neurons is similar. Like MAO-B inhibitors, COMT inhibitors slow the breakdown of dopamine in the brain, thereby improving the amount of dopamine available to neurons in the substantia nigra (Figure 12). When used with levodopa, COMT inhibitors can shorten "off" episodes by increasing on time.

Figure 12 COMT Inhibitors Help Maintain Dopamine Supply.

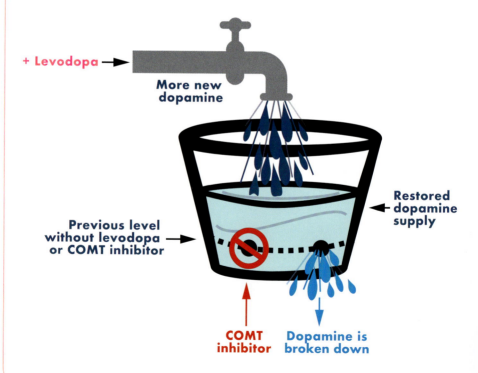

PARKINSON'S DISEASE & TREATMENTS

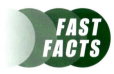

There are more than 10 million people living with Parkinson's disease worldwide. In the United States, as many as 1 million people live with Parkinson's, which is more than the combined number of people with multiple sclerosis, muscular dystrophy, and amyotrophic lateral sclerosis. Approximately 60,000 Americans are diagnosed with PD each year. This number does not reflect the thousands of cases that go undetected.

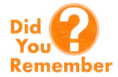

There are 3 basic ways medicines seek to correct the low dopamine levels in people with Parkinson's:
- Increase the amount available
- Provide the brain with an acceptable substitute
- Slow down dopamine elimination

Unlike MAO-B inhibitors, COMT inhibitors do not work if they are taken alone. They must be taken with levodopa.

Life With **PARKINSON'S**

Motor Symptoms & Medicines

Other medicines for treating motor symptoms

Amantadine

Amantadine was originally used as a flu treatment in the 1960s. At that time, people with PD taking amantadine also noticed a decrease in tremors. Although it is not fully known how amantadine works in Parkinson's, motor symptom control is quickly evident after a dose is taken. In recent years, amantadine has also been found useful in reducing dyskinesias that occur in people with Parkinson's taking levodopa. **In 2017, an extended-release form of amantadine was the first medicine approved by the FDA specifically to treat dyskinesia in Parkinson's.**

Adenosine A_{2a} antagonists

One of the newest medicines to treat PD motor symptoms, called **istradefylline**, belongs to the family of adenosine A_{2a} antagonists. They work by blocking a chemical in the brain called adenosine, an action that can reduce "off" periods resulting from long-term treatment with levodopa. This medicine is used as an add-on treatment to carbidopa/levodopa.

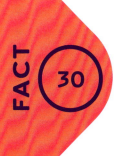

FACT 30

To address motor symptoms, other medicines people with Parkinson's may take, in addition to carbidopa/levodopa, include dopamine agonists, MAO-B inhibitors, COMT inhibitors, or an adenosine receptor antagonist.

PARKINSON'S DISEASE & TREATMENTS

What is acetylcholine?

There is a normal balance in the brain between dopamine and another neurotransmitter called acetylcholine (ACh) that can influence motor symptoms. When dopamine levels fall in people with PD, this balance is disrupted (Figure 13). Restoring this balance can improve motor symptoms.

Figure 13 Balancing Act Between Dopamine and Acetylcholine Can Influence Motor Symptoms.

Normal balance between ACh and DA

Neurotransmitter imbalance when DA is depleted in PD
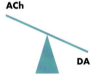

Medicine to increase DA and lower ACh action can restore balance
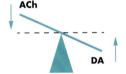

DA, dopamine
ACh, acetylcholine

Anticholinergic medicine blocks the effect of ACh. They were more commonly used in the past to treat motor symptoms of PD. This class of medicines may be used for controlling tremors, but they have many side effects, many of which are especially bothersome to older people with Parkinson's.

Amantadine is the only oral medicine that has been shown to decrease peak-dose dyskinesia in people with Parkinson's without worsening other PD symptoms.

FACT 31

Life With **PARKINSON'S**

Understanding Treatment Approaches for Motor Symptoms (Devices & Surgery)

Device- & surgery-aided Parkinson's therapies

A growing number of Parkinson's treatment options involve the use of medical devices as well as surgical options. **Device-aided Parkinson therapies** include **levodopa/carbidopa intestinal gel (LCIG) infusion** and **deep brain stimulation (DBS)**, which also has a surgical component. Ablative surgery is a purely surgical option. These additional approaches may offer effective strategies to counteract motor fluctuations and dyskinesia described earlier in this section. The choice of device-aided therapy is made by people with Parkinson's and their doctor, based on their specific medical condition, symptoms, and personal preferences.

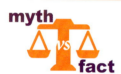

MYTH: "Parkinson's research is stalled."

FACT: It may seem as though scientists have come to a dead end; however, several recent breakthroughs regarding the delivery of PD medicines, as well as electrical brain stimulation, have occurred. According to researchers, these new developments should translate to actual clinical results in the next few years.

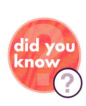

At this time, a new PD medical device is in late-stage development that aims to provide continuous **apomorphine** (page 64) via a subcutaneous **infusion** pump. If approved by the FDA, this novel treatment approach would be used for the continuous treatment of "on-off episodes" (page 59) in adults with PD who continue to experience motor symptoms after treatment with oral levodopa, and at least 1 other noninvasive Parkinson's therapy.

PARKINSON'S DISEASE & TREATMENTS

Levodopa/carbidopa intestinal gel (LCIG) infusion: This option provides levodopa infusion directly into the intestinal tract, leading to a sustained "on" episode (Figure 9). This infusion requires surgically placing a special tube through the skin, the abdomen, and the wall of the stomach. Once in place, the other end of the tube is attached to an infusion pump that is worn.

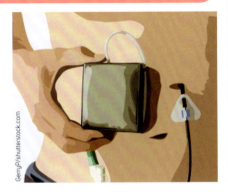

Each cassette of medicine provides up to 16 hours of continuous levodopa infusion. The pump cannot be worn when showering, bathing, or swimming. People using this device may experience similar side effects of conventional levodopa therapy in addition to higher rates of depression or falling asleep suddenly during the day.

Deep brain stimulation (DBS): Similar to levodopa, DBS can improve symptoms in certain people with Parkinson's while improving motor fluctuations. DBS involves surgically placing wires (electrodes) into a specific area of the brain along with an impulse-generating battery under the collar bone. Once turned "ON," the electric impulses delivered to the brain improve certain motor symptoms.

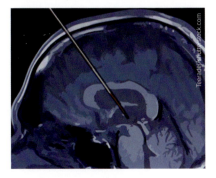

To be eligible for DBS, individuals must have had PD for at least 4 years including persistent motor complications (significant off time or dyskinesia) despite taking medicines for PD. **Cognitive function** should be as close to normal as possible because DBS can negatively impact those who have impaired thinking or memory.

Life With **PARKINSON'S**

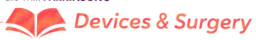

Devices & Surgery

DBS benefits
Once implanted, DBS can noticeably improve symptoms such as tremor, rigidity, stiffness, and bradykinesia. These benefits have been documented to last indefinitely, although the magnitude of benefits decreases over time. Some people with PD who undergo DBS may also be able to decrease the dose of their Parkinson's medicines. Reducing medicine doses can reduce side effects.

DBS side effects
As with any procedure, there are some risks associated with DBS surgery. Stroke, bleeding, infection, or seizures are all possible with any type of brain surgery. Following the procedure, there is a possibility that spoken words will be unclear or slurred. There is also a risk that the procedure can possibly lower cognitive abilities, which is why cognitive function should be normal or near normal to qualify for DBS.

Ablative surgery: This purely surgical procedure locates, targets, and then ablates or destroys a targeted area of the brain. The aim of this surgery is to destroy tissue that produces abnormal chemical or electrical impulses causing symptoms, while leaving the surrounding areas in the brain untouched. The most common ablative surgery for PD is **pallidotomy**, which ablates a small region of the **globus pallidus** to improve tremor, rigidity, or dyskinesias for some people with PD.

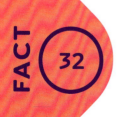

FACT 32

Similar to levodopa, deep brain stimulation (DBS) can improve symptoms in certain people with Parkinson's while improving motor fluctuations.

PARKINSON'S DISEASE & TREATMENTS

Summary: Treating motor symptoms

Options
For people with PD, a growing list of treatment options are available for motor symptoms that range from mild to hard to control. Each of the options (or combinations of options) described here are used to control motor symptoms while causing the fewest side effects possible. Because PD is a lifelong condition, you may need one or more of the treatments discussed.

Medicine and Monitoring
Once you start taking medicine for Parkinson's, it is important to monitor how well it works. All medicines should be taken on time to minimize "off" episodes and other motor symptoms, but also to ensure predictability of response and determine if a pattern emerges that may require changes in treatment.

Keeping a Symptom Diary
It may help to keep a symptom diary, particularly after you have had a PD-related surgical procedure, started using a new PD device, or after your Parkinson's medicine has been changed. You can use this diary to note any noticeable changes in your condition or side effects. Bringing your diary to different appointments can help members of your treatment team understand how any changes are impacting your functional expectations of daily living. This helps to make sure you are receiving the best treatment for your symptoms and that you experience the least amount of side effects possible.

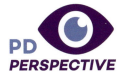

"Courage doesn't always roar. Sometimes courage is the quiet voice at the end of the day saying, 'I will try again tomorrow'."
–Mary Anne Radmacher

Overview of Non-Motor Symptoms & Approaches

As discussed briefly in section 1, there are many PD-related non-motor symptoms that can affect functional expectations of daily living. For many, these "invisible symptoms" are as distressing, or maybe more distressing, than motor deficits. Further discussed in greater detail below are those non-motor symptoms with an added focus on how their existence may be connected to PD. Included in this section are approaches (treatment) for non-motor symptoms highlighted as *"what to do about"* them. Just as with motor symptoms and related treatments, it is important that you maintain regular contact with your **health care team** to discuss any changes in non-motor symptoms or any new symptoms that you experience.

Cognitive symptoms

Most people with PD will experience cognitive changes during the course of their illness. These may include feelings of distraction, disorganization, and difficulty planning or accomplishing tasks. Your family and friends also might be able to tell you about symptoms they have observed. One cause for these problems is a low level of dopamine in the brain—the same thing that causes motor symptoms. Other brain changes may also be involved. For example, scientists are studying 2 other "messengers," acetylcholine (page 71) and **norepinephrine**, as possible additional causes of some cognitive symptoms in PD. Finally, stress, depression, and certain medicines related to having PD can also contribute.

FACT 33 One cause of cognitive symptoms is the low level of dopamine in the brains of individuals with PD—the same condition that causes motor symptoms.

PARKINSON'S DISEASE & TREATMENTS

Examples of PD-related cognitive symptoms include changes in:
- [ ] Attention
- [ ] Executive function
- [ ] Language
- [ ] Memory
- [ ] Mental processing speed

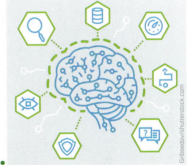

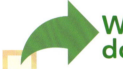

COGNITIVE SYMPTOMS

Discuss any cognitive symptoms with your health care providers, who may need to make changes to your medicines or refer you to a **neuropsychologist** for further assessment. They also might refer you to an **occupational therapist** to help you find strategies for adapting and coping.

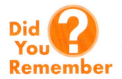

Non-motor symptoms are sometimes called "invisible symptoms."

Life With **PARKINSON'S**

Non-Motor Symptoms & Approaches

Depression

Everyone feels sad from time to time, including individuals with PD. In fact, a period of grief in reaction to a PD diagnosis is normal. Depression is different from temporary sadness, however; it is persistent, lasting for weeks or longer. Similar to cognitive changes, depression may be part of PD itself, resulting from changes in brain chemistry. For example, PD affects the areas of the brain that produce dopamine, norepinephrine, and **serotonin**—the chemical "messengers" involved in regulating mood, energy, motivation, appetite, and sleep (page 90). Other causes of depression in PD may include the significant stress of coping with a chronic illness and, potentially, side effects from medicines.

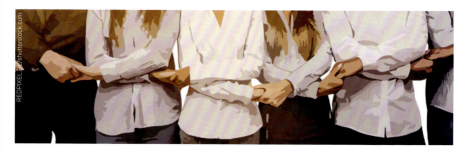

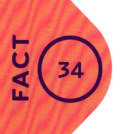

FACT 34

If you have feelings of depression, **you are not alone**. Nearly 50% of people with PD experience depression at some point during their disease course. Depression is well understood by PD health care providers and is treatable. Talk to your doctor if you are experiencing depression.

PARKINSON'S DISEASE & TREATMENTS

Examples of symptoms of depression

Depression can look different from person to person, and it can range in severity from mild to severe. Although people experience depression individually, some symptoms are common:

- Persistent sadness
- Loss of interest in activities once enjoyed
- Increased fatigue, lack of energy
- Feelings of guilt, self-criticism, worthlessness
- Change in appetite or eating habits (either poor appetite or overeating)
- Decreased attention to hygiene
- Ignoring medical and or health needs

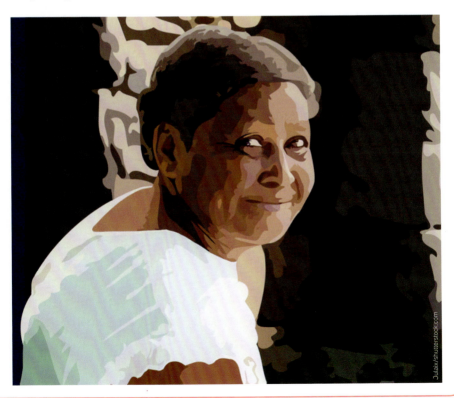

Life With **PARKINSON'S**

Non-Motor Symptoms & Approaches

Anxiety

Anxiety is less well understood than depression in PD, but it is nearly as common. People with poorly controlled anxiety often avoid social situations, to the detriment of family and work relationships. Anxiety can also interfere with memory storage, disrupt attention and the performance of complex tasks, and trigger insomnia. Interestingly, successful treatment of anxiety can reverse some of these problems.

Examples of symptoms of anxiety

- ☐ Excessive worrying
- ☐ New or intensified fears
- ☐ Uncontrollable or unwanted thoughts
- ☐ Sudden waves of terror
- ☐ Physical symptoms
    - Problems falling or staying asleep
    - Pounding heart
    - Sweating

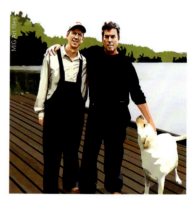

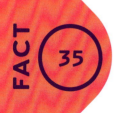

FACT 35

The successful treatment of anxiety can reverse some of its related negative effects, including insomnia, memory storage issues, disrupted attention, and challenges with the performance of complex tasks.

PARKINSON'S DISEASE & TREATMENTS

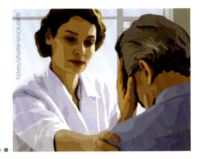

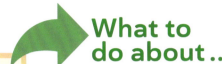

DEPRESSION & ANXIETY

As with all non-motor symptoms, talk to your health care provider. Being diagnosed is a critical first step toward effective treatment and recovery from depression and anxiety. However, many people with PD remain undiagnosed because they do not recognize that they have a mood problem or are unable to describe their symptoms. **Asking a caregiver or loved one if he or she has noticed any changes in your mood may be helpful.**

Treatments for depression and anxiety are as diverse as the symptoms and generally fall into 2 main categories: medicine and/or psychological counseling. Often, a combination of these approaches is most effective. **Treating depression is one of the most significant ways to decrease disability and improve quality of life in people with PD.**

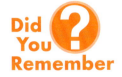

Anxiety can contribute to insomnia.

Life With **PARKINSON'S**

Non-Motor Symptoms & Approaches

PD psychosis (PDP)

The term *psychosis* may be intimidating to some. Psychosis is defined as a loss of touch with reality that can be brought on by illness, medicine, substance use, extreme stress, trauma, or a combination of these triggers. *It is not a disease in and of itself.* As discussed in section 1, PD-related psychosis can manifest as delusions (false beliefs), hallucinations (seeing things that aren't there), and other symptoms. Most hallucinations are fleeting and nonthreatening. Of note, hallucinations in people with Parkinson's are most often a side effect of medicine and not necessarily a sign of cognitive decline.

Examples of symptoms of PDP

- [ ] Delusions
- [ ] Hallucinations
- [ ] Incoherent speech
- [ ] Agitation

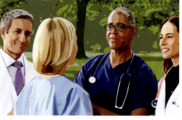

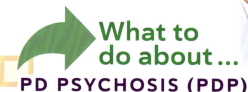

What to do about... PD PSYCHOSIS (PDP)

It is important to report any delusions or hallucinations—even if they are not bothersome—to your medical team. Treating PDP is a multistep process of identifying underlying causes and figuring out how best to address them. Typically, treatment involves adjusting medicine and/or referral to counseling.

PARKINSON'S DISEASE & TREATMENTS

50 FACTS & MORE

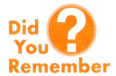 **Did You Remember** Hallucinations are most often a side effect of medicine and not necessarily a sign of cognitive decline.

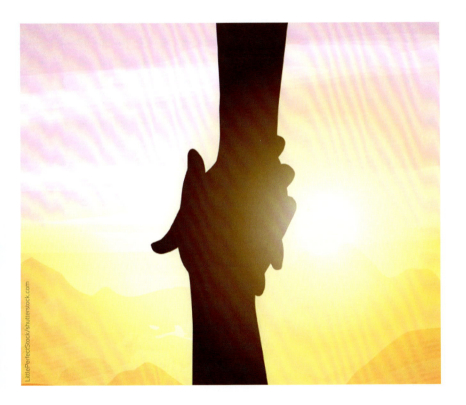

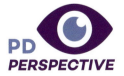 **PD PERSPECTIVE** "Hard times don't create heroes. It is during the hard times when the 'hero' within us is revealed."
–Bob Riley

Non-Motor Symptoms & Approaches

Impulse control disorders (ICDs)

Between 10% to 15% of people with PD develop ICDs while receiving dopamine-replacement therapy. Surgical treatments such as DBS may also trigger ICDs. These disorders can be upsetting and surprising to family and friends, as the behaviors may be highly out of character for the individual and can even be dangerous or costly. Not surprisingly, ICDs can place significant stress on homelife and marriage.

Examples of ICDs in people with PD

- Compulsive
    - Computer usage (internet)
    - Gambling, in person and online
    - Shopping
- Hoarding
- Hypersexuality

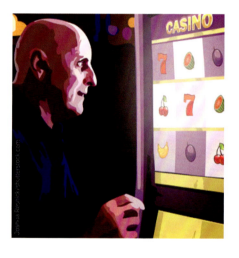

did you know?

Hypersexuality is an excessive preoccupation with sexual fantasies, urges, or behaviors that is difficult to control; causes you distress; or negatively affects your health, job, relationships, or other parts of your life. In people with PD, hypersexuality is often related to dopamine-replacement therapy. It is considered both an ICD as well as a sexual dysfunction (page 100).

PARKINSON'S DISEASE & TREATMENTS

What to do about...
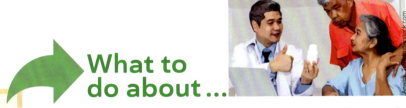

IMPULSE CONTROL DISORDERS (ICDs)

If you find yourself engaging in any of these behaviors or doing things that you feel guilty about, don't keep it to yourself. Talk to your health care team and your family right away. If the behavior is caused by a medicine, your doctor might reduce the amount or switch you to a different medicine. You may be referred to a psychotherapist or psychiatrist who will help you identify any cues that trigger the urge to engage in compulsive behaviors like gambling or shopping, and then identify actions you can take to deal with those urges. People with ICDs may also benefit from connecting with a **social worker** who can refer them to specific support groups that deal with ICDs.

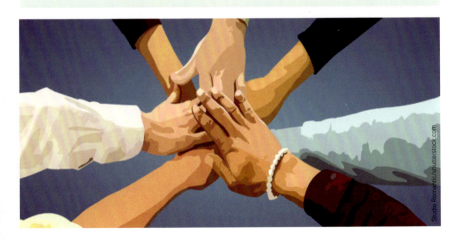

Life With PARKINSON'S
Non-Motor Symptoms & Approaches

Pseudobulbar affect (PBA)

PBA is described as random outbursts of crying or laughing that do not match the situation or the person's true feelings. Episodes are usually brief but intense and may occur several times per day. PBA can occur with a variety of neurologic diseases, including PD, that affect the areas of the brain that influence emotional expression. Disrupted signal transmissions in these areas cause PBA. According to PBA Info, about 24% of people with PD may exhibit PBA during the course of their illness.

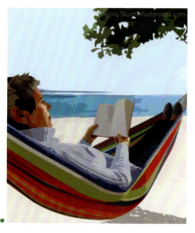

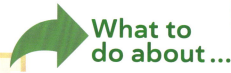

What to do about... PSEUDOBULBAR AFFECT (PBA)

Discuss the behavior with your health care providers. They can provide personalized recommendations for you. They may suggest lifestyle strategies such as tracking what usually triggers your PBA episodes and trying to avoid those triggers. Awareness, breathing, and relaxation may also help. For example, when you feel PBA approaching, it may be helpful to try to focus on something else, shift your body to a different posture, and take slow deep breaths while relaxing your body as much as possible until you are back in control.

50 FACTS & MORE

PARKINSON'S DISEASE & TREATMENTS

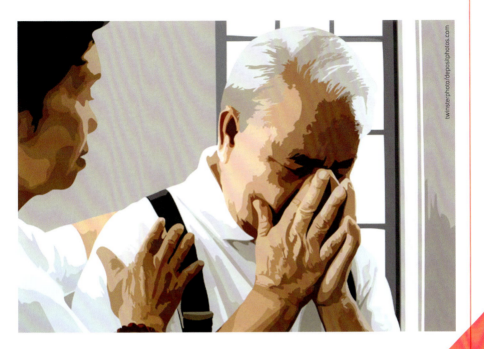

PBA can be mistaken for depression; however, episodes of PBA often do not *match* the situation or the person's feelings. People with PBA may be happy about something, but then without warning, start sobbing; or they may laugh loudly in an inappropriate situation.

FACT 36

Life With **PARKINSON'S**

Non-Motor Symptoms & Approaches

Neurogenic orthostatic hypotension (NOH)
Neurogenic orthostatic hypotension is common in PD. It occurs when the nervous system loses its ability to regulate blood pressure as a person stands up from a sitting or lying position. Blood pressure drops quickly, causing symptoms such as lightheadedness upon standing in about 20% of people with Parkinson's. Additional symptoms that may be present include: cognitive difficulties, fatigue, visual disturbance, or falls. These symptoms can be improved by getting up slowly from a reclined position, drinking more fluids, adding more salt to meals, and, if at all possible, using thigh-high compressive leg stockings. Medicine may also be needed, including one or more of the following: **droxidopa**, **fludrocortisone**, or **midodrine**.

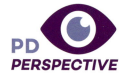

"Impossible is just a big word thrown around by small men who find it easier to live in the world they've been given than to explore the power they have to change it. Impossible is not a fact. It's an opinion. Impossible is not a declaration. It's a dare. Impossible is potential. Impossible is temporary. Impossible is nothing."
–Muhammad Ali

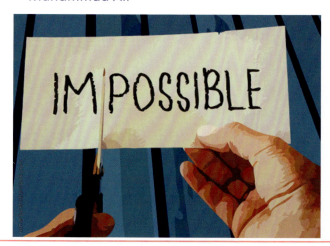

50 FACTS & MORE

PARKINSON'S DISEASE & TREATMENTS

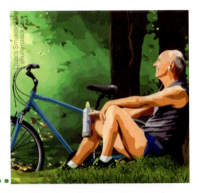

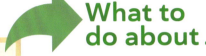

What to do about... NEUROGENIC ORTHOSTATIC HYPOTENSION

Talk to your doctor immediately if you experience lightheadedness or feel dizzy when sitting or standing up. Together, you may do a medicine review to identify potentially problematic medicines you are taking, and reduce or replace them. You may also be encouraged to move more slowly when rising and engage in physical exercise to strengthen your body or avoid weakening. Importantly, you will want to reduce your risk for falls and injury. Medicine for NOH is available. Your doctor may prescribe droxidopa, fludrocortisone, or midodrine—sometimes in combination.

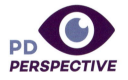

"Always remember you are braver than you believe, stronger than you seem, smarter than you think and twice as beautiful as you've ever imagined."
–Dr. Seuss

Life With **PARKINSON'S**

Non-Motor Symptoms & Approaches

Sleep problems

Poor sleep and impaired daytime alertness are some of the most common symptoms affecting people with PD. In fact, most will experience sleep-related problems at some point after diagnosis. Two common and sometimes related sleep disorders that affect people with Parkinson's are insomnia and excessive daytime sleepiness (EDS). Insomnia is defined as repeated difficulty falling asleep, staying asleep, or getting good quality of sleep, causing daytime sleepiness. People with PD usually fall asleep without much trouble but wake up frequently throughout the night and have trouble falling back to sleep. EDS is the inability to maintain wakefulness or alertness during the day, often due to lack of proper sleep at night. Problems sleeping at night, or staying alert during the day can have negative effects on quality of life and serious safety implications (for example, driving).

There are several underlying causes for PD-related sleep problems. For example, the changes in the brain that lead to PD-related motor symptoms can affect the **sleep-wake cycle**. **Vivid dreams**, an occasional side effect of levodopa-based medicine, can disturb sleep as can difficulty getting comfortable, whether from pain or not being able to roll over in bed. In addition, as mentioned in section 1, people with PD often have nocturia, excessive urination at night. Getting up frequently to go to the bathroom can stop you from sleeping soundly.

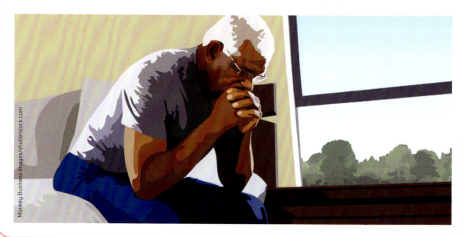

PARKINSON'S DISEASE & TREATMENTS

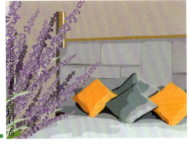

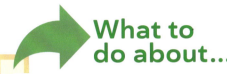# SLEEP PROBLEMS

If you are experiencing sleep problems, try improving your sleep hygiene. If the problems persist, tell your health care provider. He or she will talk to you about strategies to help you sleep better. This could include prescribing sleep medicine or recommending a sleep specialist.

What is sleep hygiene?
Similar to practicing a dental hygiene regimen to encourage good oral health (for example, brushing your teeth, flossing), practicing sleep hygiene is one of the most straightforward ways to promote consistent, uninterrupted sleep. The practice involves many different elements that can be customized to the individual. Some methods include keeping a consistent sleep schedule (waking up and going to bed at the same time each day), making your bedroom comfortable and free of disruptions, following a relaxing pre-bed routine, and building healthy habits during the day.

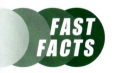 If pain interferes with your sleep, talk to your doctor as soon as you can. Do not wait.

Life With **PARKINSON'S**

Non-Motor Symptoms & Approaches

Pain
With so many different symptoms affecting people with PD, pain sometimes is overlooked. However, ongoing untreated pain can have negative effects on your quality of life and daily functioning. In fact, between 40% to 80% of people with PD report experiencing some form of pain during the course of their illness, and for many it's one of the most troubling non-motor symptoms. As discussed in section 1 (pages 34-35), people with PD may experience 5 types of pain.

Examples of PD-related pain syndromes (described on pages 34 and 35)

- [ ] Musculoskeletal
- [ ] Dystonic (related to muscle contractions)
- [ ] Nerve
- [ ] Central (related to damaged **central nervous system [CNS]**)
- [ ] Depression-related pain

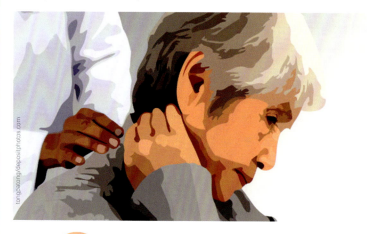

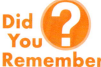 Chronic pain and depression may be connected. If a person experiences depression, it may worsen pain as well as other PD symptoms, such as insomnia.

50 FACTS & MORE

PARKINSON'S DISEASE & TREATMENTS

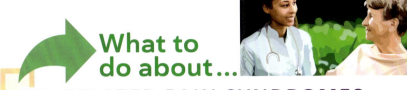

What to do about...
PD-RELATED PAIN SYNDROMES

As with other aspects of PD, each person will have an individual journey to discover the best way to treat their pain, but the first step is a familiar one: Speak with your health care team right away. Together you will work to understand the underlying cause of your pain and explore the wide array of treatment options. Pain management takes many forms, including non-medical, behavioral, lifestyle interventions, and/or introduction to several different types of pain medicine.

Lots of people are embarrassed to bring up certain topics with their doctor—from changes in feelings and mood, to sexual dysfunction, to incontinence or problems controlling saliva. However, these are common subjects in PD, as they are related to the disease process itself as well as side effects from medicine. Nothing should be considered off limits in discussions with your health care team. The more you talk about these issues, the less embarrassing they become. Your doctor has heard it all!

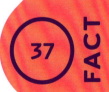

FACT 37

Life With **PARKINSON'S**

Non-Motor Symptoms & Approaches

Constipation

Constipation is considered by many experts to be a core symptom of PD. It occurs in 80% to 90% of people with PD, and may start becoming a problem even before the onset of motor symptoms like tremor and stiffness. Constipation is defined as an alteration in stool frequency, consistency, and/or passage of stool. PD affects muscles and nerves in the gastrointestinal tract, slowing down the time it takes for the stomach to empty and for material to move through the intestines. This is referred to as a "slow gut." Constipation in PD can be debilitating.

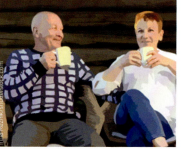

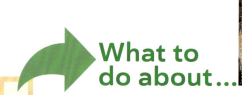

What to do about... PD-RELATED CONSTIPATION

Effective strategies for reducing PD-related constipation include getting as much vigorous daily exercise as possible and drinking 6 to 8 glasses of water each day. Having grains with dried fruit or dates in the morning along with a strong cup of coffee can also encourage morning bowel movements. Importantly, avoid using Metamucil or other forms of psyllium because these products tend to become hard in the slow gut and end up actually making constipation worse. If these efforts do not provide relief, ask your health care provider about other strategies including available medicines.

PARKINSON'S DISEASE & TREATMENTS

Bladder issues

Bladder issues may appear later in the course of PD. The most common problems are the need to urinate often (frequency) and the need to urinate immediately (urgency). These symptoms usually indicate that your bladder is telling your brain that it is full and needs to empty when, in fact, it is not. This can happen at any time, so you might have to get up multiple times during the night to go to the bathroom (nocturia). As noted above, this can interfere with your ability to sleep soundly.

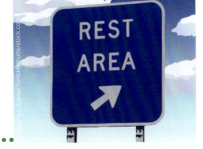

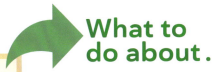

BLADDER ISSUES

If urinary problems persist, or other urinary changes occur, talk to your doctors. They will want to determine whether the problem is related to PD or another cause, such as a bladder or **urinary tract infection**, **enlarged prostate**, or other medical issue. In addition to lifestyle adjustments, medicines are available to help with bladder issues. Your doctor may also refer you to a bladder specialist (**urologist**).

Life With **PARKINSON'S**

Non-Motor Symptoms & Approaches

Speech & voice problems

Some people with PD-related speech and voice problems are reluctant to participate in conversation and feel a lack of confidence in social settings. This can greatly diminish quality of life and social interaction. The causes of speech and voice impairment in PD usually involve muscle-related motor symptoms and/or changes in speech-related brain signal transmissions (page 44).

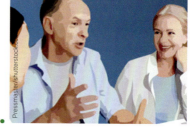

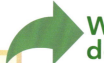

What to do about...
SPEECH & VOICE PROBLEMS

Tell your doctors if you experience any changes in your speech or voice, or if your loved ones have mentioned such changes to you. Early changes may not be easily detected, but the sooner you get a speech evaluation and start speech therapy, the more effective it can be.

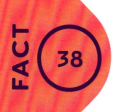

FACT 38

Speech disorders can progressively diminish quality of life for a person with PD. Early speech evaluation and speech therapy lead to a greater likelihood of regaining and retaining communication skills.

50 FACTS & MORE

PARKINSON'S DISEASE & TREATMENTS

 People with PD may not be aware that their speech is getting softer. When they are asked to bring their voice to normal loudness, they may feel as if they are shouting.

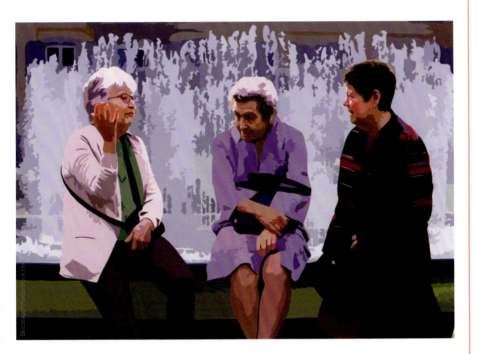

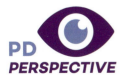

"Act as if what you do makes a difference. It does."
—William James

Life With **PARKINSON'S**

Non-Motor Symptoms & Approaches

Sialorrhea

Excessive drooling, called sialorrhea, can be a symptom of advanced PD, particularly during "off" episodes. Symptoms can range from mild wetting of the pillow during sleep to embarrassing outpourings of saliva. The cause of excessive drooling in PD may be connected to a reduction in the body's ability to maintain autonomic functions, such as swallowing. It may also be connected to the slowing and stiffening of muscles around the jaw that may occur in people with Parkinson's. Although the amount of saliva your body produces is normal, swallowing less often or incompletely can lead to an inability to manage the flow of saliva in and around the mouth.

 April is Parkinson's Awareness Month.

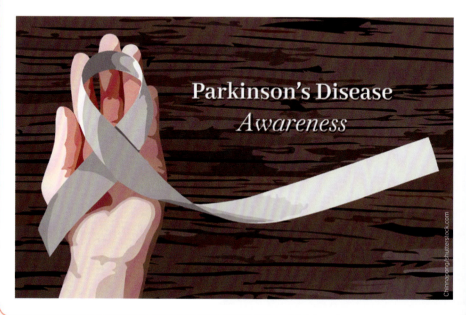

PARKINSON'S DISEASE & TREATMENTS

What to do about...
SIALORRHEA

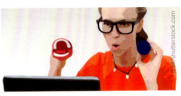

Talk to your doctors if you have problems with drooling. They may refer you to a **speech-language therapist** who can perform a swallow test to diagnose any difficulties and provide strategies to help reduce drooling. One temporary method is to suck on hard candy or chew gum (preferably sugarless). This activates the jaw and automatic swallowing reflex, helping to clear saliva. Another is to wear a sweatband on your forearm or wrist to discretely wipe your mouth when needed. If these lifestyle strategies are not effective, your doctor may adjust your medicine to improve your ability to swallow. A number of therapies are available for the treatment of sialorrhea, including oral and injectable medicines. Ask your health care provider if there is one that is right for you.

FACT 39

Drooling, swallowing issues, and speech problems are considered to be non-motor PD symptoms, even though they are related to poor coordination, bradykinesia (slow movements), and rigidity in muscles of the mouth and throat.

Life With **PARKINSON'S**

Non-Motor Symptoms & Approaches

Sexual dysfunction

Sex is a natural part of the adult human experience, and people living with PD may face concerns about their ability to have and enjoy sex as the disease progresses. PD-related sexual dysfunction is common. Physical immobility in bed, sleep disturbances, depression, and changes in thinking can affect sexual desire in men and women. Men may also experience erectile dysfunction, and women may experience decreased sex drive or pain with intercourse. Causes include PD itself, which involves the loss of dopamine, the principal "messenger" of reward and pleasure in the brain; psychological changes related to decreased positive body image; and side effects of various PD medicines. Hypersexuality also can occur in some people taking dopamine agonists, as well as for some on higher doses of levodopa (page 84).

Examples of symptoms of PD-related sexual dysfunction

- ☐ Decreased sex drive
- ☐ Painful intercourse
- ☐ Erectile dysfunction

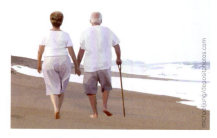

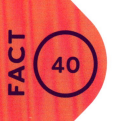

FACT 40

It's important to realize that non-motor symptoms are quite common. Research shows that some people actually develop PD-related non-motor symptoms like depression and sleep problems *years* before they get a PD diagnosis.

PARKINSON'S DISEASE & TREATMENTS

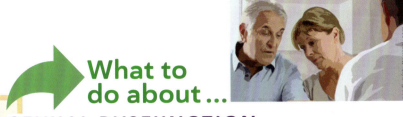

What to do about...
SEXUAL DYSFUNCTION

Do not be embarrassed to talk with your doctor about issues of sexual health and satisfaction. He or she will help you find solutions best suited to your individual circumstances. A common approach is decreasing or stopping medicines that may be causing the problem. For hypersexuality related to dopamine replacement therapy, decreasing the dose or discontinuation of dopamine agonists can resolve what is essentially an ICD. Discussing the situation with your partner is also important. People with PD can have healthy sexual relationships, but open communication with your partner, doctor, and perhaps a therapist are key to finding solutions.

did you know?

There are many holistic approaches to living well with Parkinson's. Physical, mental, and spiritual therapeutic approaches used by people with Parkinson's include:

- Yoga
- Massage
- Acupuncture
- Dance
- Tai chi
- Meditation

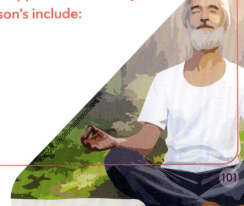

Keywords & Concepts Introduced in Section 3*

- ✔ Activities of daily living (ADL)
- ✔ Advance directive
- ✔ American Medical Association (AMA)
- ✔ American Parkinson's Disease Association
- ✔ Americans With Disabilities Act (ADA)
- ✔ Autonomic nervous system
- ✔ Caregiver Action Network
- ✔ Caregiver Self-Assessment Questionnaire
- ✔ Caring.com
- ✔ Dietitian
- ✔ Driver rehabilitation specialist
- ✔ Electronic banking
- ✔ Estate planning
- ✔ European Parkinson's Disease Association (EPDA)
- ✔ Family Caregiver Alliance (FCA)
- ✔ Financial plan
- ✔ Flexible spending accounts
- ✔ Geriatrician
- ✔ Health care proxy
- ✔ Home health aide
- ✔ Human resources (HR)
- ✔ Long-term care insurance
- ✔ Medicaid
- ✔ Medicare
- ✔ Melvin Weinstein Parkinson's Foundation (MWPF)
- ✔ Michael J. Fox Foundation
- ✔ Mileposts
- ✔ Multidisciplinary team
- ✔ Parkinson's Foundation Caregiver Self-Assessment
- ✔ Parkinson's Foundation Helpline
- ✔ Parkinson's IQ + You
- ✔ Parkinson's Passport
- ✔ Pharmacist
- ✔ Physiotherapist
- ✔ Podiatrist
- ✔ Positivity
- ✔ Power of attorney
- ✔ Sex therapist
- ✔ Telecommuting
- ✔ The Parkinson Alliance
- ✔ Thermodysregulation
- ✔ Well Spouse Association (WSA)
- ✔ Will

*Terms listed here are addressed in this section and can be found with their definitions in the Glossary (page 196).

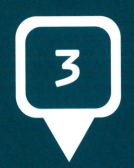

SECTION 3:
ON THE ROAD—
THE PD JOURNEY

> "It is not the strongest of the species that survive, it is the one most adaptable to change."
>
> –Charles Darwin

PARKINSON'S DISEASE:
Pack a Positive Attitude for the Trip

Following a diagnosis of Parkinson's, the natural question becomes, "**Can I still live well with the disorder?**". The answer is an emphatic yes!, although a key element of success is to maintain a positive outlook. Parkinson's takes many different courses and one person's experience may be substantially different from another's. *Positivity is key*. Symptoms that appear may come slowly to one person or change more quickly in another, but awareness of these challenges and ways in which they can be addressed are vital to maintaining emotional health—and the same is true for PD caregivers and family members. *Knowledge and preparation increase positivity*.

In this section we present common **MILEPOSTS** from **The Parkinson's Journey** in the form of *Frequently Asked Directions (FADs)*. In addition to the fairly exhaustive coverage of PD-related topics in sections 1 and 2, we asked people living with Parkinson's, "What important questions would you have asked, or asked earlier, on your own Parkinson's journey?" We also asked those with experience supporting people with PD (caregivers, movement disorder specialists, spouses) to share with us their most common questions, salient observations, and pearls of wisdom. To all such queries we have attempted to supply concise, thoughtful, well-researched responses. We would appreciate receiving additional ideas for inclusion in future updates of *Life With Parkinson's 50 Facts & More*. Please send your suggestions and comments to Mileposts@50Facts.com.

It helps to be goal-oriented by understanding that, together with the challenges that inevitably appear, short- and long-term functional goals can help mitigate the life of a person with Parkinson's. Ultimately, the path one takes along the PD journey is entirely an individual one. Symptoms, unique challenges, responses, family and caregiver assistance, medical coverage, and financial issues are experienced through the filter of one's own life. A PD life is still a life, with all the promise and fulfillment that life suggests, *and positivity will enhance that life*.

Life With **PARKINSON'S**

A Postcard From Frank C. Church:
See yourself happy*

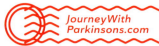

JourneyWith Parkinsons.com

"Take in Frank's Take" on living with Parkinson's: "Stay hopeful, be positive, remain persistent, because as long as you're alive, you can do it all. As always, stay focused and determined; strive for health and strength. And through it all, try to incorporate happiness into your daily life to help manage your Parkinson's."

Below is a helpful list of ACTIONS that can ACTIVATE positivity at any time during any day in the life of a person with Parkinson's. This top 10 list of things to do for positivity was created by Frank C. Church (journeywithparkinsons.com), a professor at the University of North Carolina and a person with Parkinson's.

STAY IN THE PRESENT MOMENT: Life is constantly moving. Your Parkinson's is always present, and yes it's a nuisance. Being able to focus on the current moment, whether good or bad, hard or easy, is better; don't complicate the thought by dwelling on yesterday, tomorrow, or your disorder. Try to stay in the present.

GO FOR A WALK OUTSIDE: Stretch frequently and exercise daily if possible. For people with Parkinson's, exercise is essential and beneficial. And it only takes 20 minutes to achieve some benefit.

EAT BETTER and your body will be happier: We all know, you are what you eat. Your body, your mind, and your battle with Parkinson's will benefit if you carve out time to eat better.

PRACTICE MINDFUL MEDITATION even 5 minutes will make a difference. In managing Parkinson's, we should work to release/relieve mental stress. Meditation reduces stress and allows us to become more mindful. Simply stated, meditation creates in you a stress-free, relaxed, and happy place.

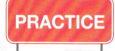

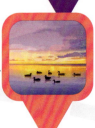

50 FACTS & MORE

 DO SOMETHING NICE FOR SOMEONE ELSE: Be kind to others, you'll feel better. Doing something nice for someone else reminds you that you're human; the happy feeling should momentarily put your Parkinson's behind shutters.

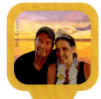

 SMILE MORE: It just matters to smile, get out behind the "Parkinson's mask." Smile big, smile more, keep trying.

SHARE SOME CHOCOLATE: Occasionally ignoring "eat better"–*across the page here* is ok, as chocolate falls into a uniquely sinful class of food.

PRACTICE GRATITUDE: Be thankful for what you have today. Be thankful for your career, your life, your partner, your support team, even your hot coffee. Practice gratitude to help soothe passing moments of pain, doubt, or difficulty. Express your gratitude to family/friends/loved ones; they will in turn be grateful.

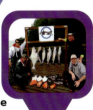

SLEEP MORE: Sleep repairs/rejuvenates our bodies and minds. Sleep renews our daily lease on life to begin again. For those of us with Parkinson's, we must always keep trying to get more sleep.

LISTEN TO A SONG or watch a YouTube music video: Sing along, recall a happy memory, focus on the beat, get up and dance.

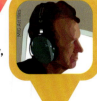

*Adapted with permission from Frank C. Church.

Life With **PARKINSON'S**

 # Me & My Parkinson's

PD & Me

 I am overwhelmed with my diagnosis. What now? How do I get and stay organized?

 The most important steps you can take are to seek help right from the beginning and commit to increasing your PD-related health literacy (page 42) to understand as much as you can about PD and the journey ahead. Support and education will help you deal with current and future PD-related challenges. Planning well, and then taking action early will enable you to understand and deal with the many effects of the disease.

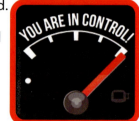

Strategies can be designed to help you regain a sense of control over your life and improve your quality of life.

Steps you can take when feeling overwhelmed include the following:

- Communicate with friends and family about your PD. Don't isolate yourself. Your friends and family will want to help you

- Continue to focus on and be involved in activities you enjoy

- Make it a habit to ask your doctor, nurse, or other health care provider to repeat any instructions or medical terms that you don't understand or remember. Make sure you understand how your health care providers are best available to respond to additional questions or concerns that may come up

- Identify and make use of resources and support services offered locally, including the hospital or support groups in your community

Frequently Asked Directions Along the Journey

 Will my diagnosis of PD reduce my life span?

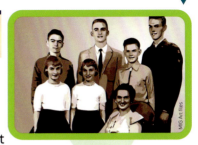

 Nowadays, according to research, people with Parkinson's can expect to live nearly as long as those without the disorder. Parkinson's is not fatal, and the key to living a long life is early detection and addressing complications as they develop. It is especially important to pay careful attention to safety issues such as falls, and to obtain the best clinical care possible.

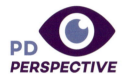 *"If you don't like the road you're walking, start paving another one."*
–Roald Dahl

 How will my PD progress?

 The Parkinson's experience can differ greatly from one person to another. For some people, tremor or falling down is the principle problem, whereas for others slowed movements or muscle rigidity is the most troublesome. Non-motor symptoms may appear 6 to 20 years before the diagnosis of PD is made, but their appearance is not sufficient for a diagnosis of PD. Some people with Parkinson's have stable disease for many years, whereas others do not. The point is, the Parkinson's journey can vary greatly and one should not have preconceived notions about its course.

Life With PARKINSON'S

Me & My Parkinson's

 Will I get all of the symptoms of PD?

 There is no accurate way to predict how your symptoms will advance. Your doctor will work to reduce the effects of any PD-related symptoms you may experience and to prevent further complications, while striving to address quality-of-life issues. Individuals with PD do not necessarily experience all the symptoms, and the severity of symptoms can vary widely. The course of this disease is famously hard to predict.

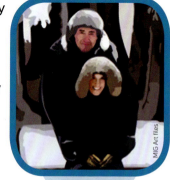

 What is the best way to tell my spouse/partner that I have Parkinson's?

 First, acknowledge that your spouse/partner has likely already noticed symptoms, so they are aware that something is amiss, although they may not know precisely what. Revealing a definitive diagnosis actually may be a relief. It may be a source of anxiety or stress to continue thinking about telling your spouse/partner about your diagnosis. It is unquestionably better, therefore, to inform the most important people in your life. Your spouse/partner will want to know as much as possible about the disease and will also start to consider how your diagnosis will affect their life. Caregiving can be seen in very different ways by different people, and feeling scared of the responsibility is not at all unusual. There are special caregiver support groups (page 117), and these can be especially helpful for elderly spouse caregivers.

Frequently Asked Directions Along the Journey

> It is important that as the person with Parkinson's, you appreciate your spouse's efforts and that you tell them so often. As you work together to increase PD-related health literacy, address symptoms, and improve your quality of life, you may find that your relationship with your spouse/partner grows stronger.

Talking with your spouse/partner about intimacy concerns may help keep this vital relationship healthy. Don't be afraid to discuss this topic with a health care provider. Remember, they have heard it all before and this is what they are there for. If necessary, they can refer you to an appropriate therapist. Of note, the Davis Phinney Foundation for Parkinson's (davisphinneyfoundation.org) has a sexual dysfunction worksheet that will guide your discussions about intimacy with your doctor.

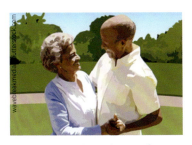

Regular communication about and within your relationships will help you to stay close and maintain openness.

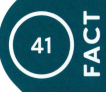

FACT 41

Life With **PARKINSON'S**

MILEPOSTS — Me & My Parkinson's

PD & Family-Social Network

What is the best way to tell family members that I have Parkinson's?

Approaches vary by age, here are some suggestions:

Experts note that often it is better to be open about one's PD diagnosis. Hiding your condition will likely fail in the long run and even very young children can sense when something is not right.

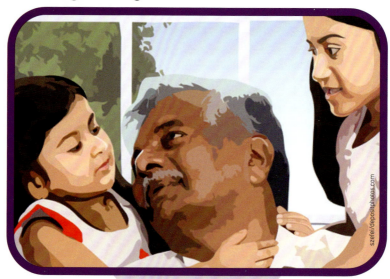

Parkinson's is best managed when everyone discusses their concerns and shares information about symptoms, quality-of-life issues, and medicines. Family and friends will be an important source of support. As the person with PD, you must continually show appreciation to this extended social group, as they help to maintain your lifestyle.

Frequently Asked Directions Along the Journey

Talking about PD with young children or grandchildren

- Trying to protect children from possibly upsetting news is a noble goal, but if done correctly children will often quickly adapt. Young children may be concerned that PD is contagious, or somehow their fault, or that you might die, but when told that none of these things is true, they often quickly pivot to the normal concerns of children

- As symptoms change or advance, children may become frustrated that you are no longer able to engage in some of their usual and favorite activities. Explaining what is happening and why you can't join in should alleviate frustration

- It is unwise to give much responsibility over your care to children, but be generous in your praise for any help they do give you

- When to explain your diagnosis and in what setting may be influenced by opportunity, but it is best to discuss PD in a calm environment with few, if any, distractions. Not every question they have needs to be answered at once. There will be plenty of time for further conversations, particularly as the symptoms of PD change

- Keep explanations as simple as possible for young children, and let their questions help guide the discussion. Medical terms should be avoided as they are too confusing. Ask them questions to make sure they have not misconstrued what you have told them

- Some children may be troubled by this news. Referring them to a therapist to further discuss your PD diagnosis may be helpful. There are specialized therapists who focus on families experiencing long-term medical conditions

Life With **PARKINSON'S**

 # Me & My Parkinson's

Talking about PD with older children and young adults

- Just as with younger children, preparation is important; the time and setting should be carefully considered

- Some older children and young adults may be concerned about caregiving roles, and may worry about your future care needs. Others may wonder what to say if friends come over and notice unusual symptoms

- Sometimes taking an older child or young adult to one of your doctor's appointments will help answer questions and serve to normalize the overall experience of your illness

Communicating with your social network, including extended family and friends

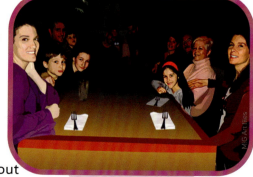

Parkinson's is best managed when everyone discusses their concerns and shares information about symptoms, quality-of-life issues, and medicines. Family and friends will be an important source of support. As the person with PD, you must continually show appreciation to this extended social group, as they help you to maintain your lifestyle.

Frequently Asked Directions Along the Journey

Additional social considerations

Social activities with your family and friends are important for emotional stability and should be continued and cherished. Just because you have PD does not mean you have to say goodbye to rewarding friendships and social interactions. By contrast, you should realize that independent activities away from your spouse/partner are recommended so you each continue your healthy independence.

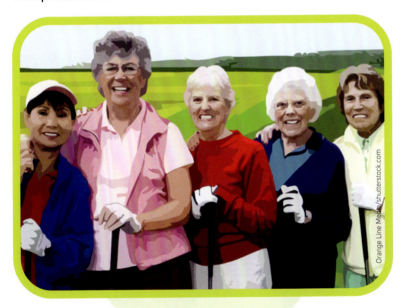

Ask your doctor about and do home research on PD support groups that may be helpful, and explore and accept any benefits that you might qualify for.

Life With **PARKINSON'S**

Me & My Parkinson's

 What about my role as a parent?

 Parenting does not end once you receive the diagnosis of Parkinson's. Nonetheless, adaptation will be needed as time passes. The key is to maintain good communication with all concerned and be prepared to make adjustments to your role over time.

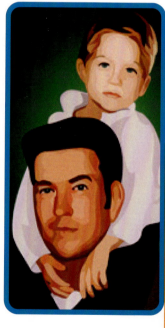

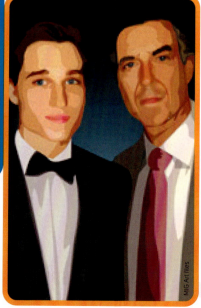

50 FACTS & MORE

Frequently Asked Directions Along the Journey

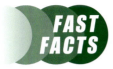
FAST FACTS

Specific sites focus on the needs of caregivers of individuals with Parkinson's. Here are 4 excellent websites to explore and share. Access the url and simply search "caregiver."

caregiver.org

hopkinsmedicine.org

michaeljfox.org

parkinson.org

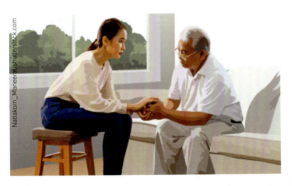

Being a PD caregiver is hard work. Caregivers need, deserve, and benefit from support.

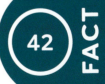

FACT 42

Life With **PARKINSON'S**

Me & My Parkinson's

PD Health Care & Safety

How do I find a doctor knowledgeable about Parkinson's disease?

The Parkinson's Foundation recommends that people with PD should find a movement disorder specialist who understands all aspects of the disease, including current treatment options and the latest research findings. People with PD should work to not only find a competent and empathetic physician but also other members of what will become a **multidisciplinary team**. Doctors should provide care as well as advice to help you negotiate the ups and downs of PD.

Specialists in PD are not evenly distributed throughout the US. If there are no such specialists in your area, then traveling to one, if affordable, once or twice a year may be an option. PD specialists might then be able to work with your local physician, preferably a neurologist, to oversee care. The Parkinson's Foundation (Parkinson.org) has an up-to-date list of US-based PD specialists.

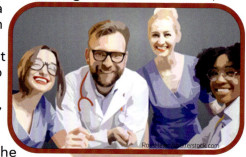

People with PD should see their doctor 2 to 4 times a year, but more often may be required if there are concerns with treatment.

50 FACTS & MORE

Frequently Asked Directions Along the Journey

 What types of health care providers might be on my PD care team?

 In the beginning, your team may not include all of these specialists, and you may never need some of them; however, each can be helpful to individuals with PD.

TEAM PARKINSON'S

- ❏ Primary care provider
- ❏ Neurologist
- ❏ **Geriatrician**
- ❏ Urologist
- ❏ **Pharmacist**
- ❏ Psychologist
- ❏ Speech-language therapist
- ❏ Occupational therapist
- ❏ Dietitian
- ❏ **Physiotherapist**
- ❏ **Podiatrist**
- ❏ **Sex therapist**
- ❏ Social worker

Life With **PARKINSON'S**

MILEPOSTS
Me & My Parkinson's

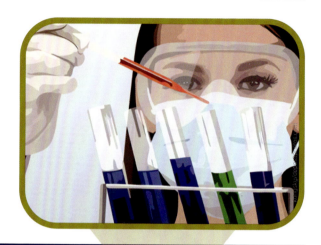

 Should I join a clinical trial?

Parkinson's disease is a major area of research. Developing effective treatments is an important goal of both the research community and the pharmaceutical industry. No advance in Parkinson's therapy has ever been found without the willingness of others to join a clinical trial.

Trials to help with Parkinson's symptoms require only that you have a diagnosis of PD. Trials to slow the progression of your disease, however, require proof that the specific experimental intervention being tested has a chance of correcting the biological abnormality that is driving your particular Parkinson's. Unfortunately, most trials today that are aimed at reducing the progression of PD are not yet able to match their specific proposed therapies to the individual people with Parkinson's most biologically suitable to benefit (see discussion on page 21). Until they are, the trials in which it is most worthy of participating in are those aimed to help with your symptoms.

50 FACTS & MORE

Frequently Asked Directions Along the Journey

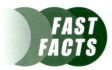 Clinical trials for Parkinson's disease can be researched by visiting the exact locations below on the following sites:

apdaparkinson.org/research/clinical-trials/

michaeljfox.org/trial-finder

michaeljfox.org/join-study

CLINICAL TRIALS

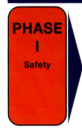 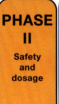

PHASE I — Safety
PHASE II — Safety and dosage
PHASE III — Safety and efficacy
PHASE IV — Post-approval surveillance

FACT 43

When a clinical trial is used to study medicines and medical devices, it is conducted in phases. The trials at each phase help scientists answer different types of questions about the medicine, therapy, or device being evaluated.

Life With **PARKINSON'S**

Me & My Parkinson's

Is deep brain stimulation (DBS) an option for me?

Not all people with Parkinson's are candidates for DBS, which is a surgical procedure. If you are interested in learning more about it, ask your doctor if, or when, you might be a candidate. As discussed on page 73, the idea of DBS is to send an electrical impulse to the part of the brain that controls motor function to gain improvement. DBS is not a cure for Parkinson's, nor does it slow progression of the disease. However, improvement in PD symptoms can last several years after DBS therapy.

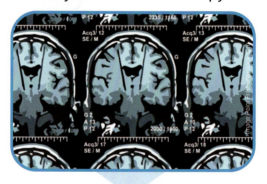

FACT 44

Survey data suggest that although DBS does not halt disease progression in PD, it provides durable symptomatic relief and allows many individuals to maintain **activities of daily living (ADLs)** over long-term follow-up for more than 10 years.

50 FACTS & MORE

Frequently Asked Directions Along the Journey

 My PD can make me feel unsteady at times. Should I be concerned about falling?

Falling is perhaps the most common and dangerous complication of PD because it can lead to fractures or head injuries. Parkinson's may impair balance and create a slow, stiff, or halting gait. Further, individuals with PD may exhibit a stooped posture, struggle with fatigue, and have low blood pressure. All of these factors increase the risk for falls. These risks are enhanced when people with Parkinson's experience freezing gait. Freezing can make elevators and negotiating crowds quite difficult.

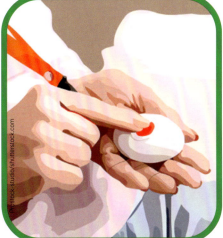

The risk for falls may be lessened by staying aware of the risk itself and using devices like canes and walkers to steady your gait. Some people with PD may benefit from gait training; others may feel steadier on their feet with a change in medicine. Accommodations in the home may be a prime consideration to avoid the risk for falling. For ideas and further information on such changes, see appendix A on page 184.

Life With **PARKINSON'S**

Me & My Parkinson's

My PD Life

Where can I connect with people like me, who are living a PD Life?

Learning from others is vital as you negotiate the physical and emotional challenges of this disease. In addition to getting advice on dealing with the physical demands you may experience, it will also be important to gain first-hand information and strategies for coping with the stresses of living with Parkinson's. You should remember that you have a physician as well as a clinical team that is concerned for your well-being. There are

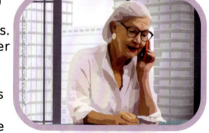

several good Parkinson's websites, including those for Parkinson's clinical associations, which have excellent resources that will help you mitigate the challenges of the PD life.

And finally, there are support groups where people can meet and share their experiences, and by so doing gain strength from their mutual stories. Some support groups have become quite sophisticated and can offer targeted educational programs covering specific demographics of people with PD—for example, younger people with Parkinson's. The Parkinson's Foundation has a list of support groups. You can email them at Helpline@Parkinson.org.

50 FACTS & MORE

Frequently Asked Directions Along the Journey

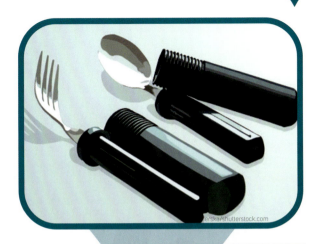

Are there devices that can help me with my PD-related eating challenges?

Tremor can disrupt the motions used in eating, which can be troublesome as these actions have been used by you for years, ergo they are deeply ingrained in your behaviors. There are solutions available such as large-grip and bendable utensils, spoons with especially deep bowls, and plates with non-slip eating surfaces and guards. Such innovations can be quite helpful in making eating less stressful.

You can find specifically designed PD-friendly eating utensils by researching the internet. Liftware is a company that offers specifically designed tableware for people with Parkinson's (liftware.com).

Life With **PARKINSON'S**

Me & My Parkinson's

 How much can weather influence my Parkinson's?

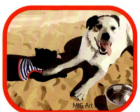

 Heat and/or cold intolerance is called **thermodysregulation**, which is an unusually big word for a condition that is not uncommon among people with PD. Cold weather can aggravate your Parkinson's symptoms, and heat intolerance can promote excessive sweating. The **autonomic nervous system** can be impaired in people with PD, and when that is the case overheating can result.

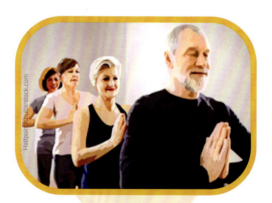

 Does stress impact my PD?

There is a definite link between stressful events and worsening of Parkinson's symptoms. The key to remember is that heightened PD symptoms will resolve once the stress has gone away. Therefore, it is very important for those with Parkinson's to actively remove stressors or work to lessen their impact.

Frequently Asked Directions Along the Journey

What is the effect of mental activity on my Parkinson's?

As we age, keeping mentally active is important for mental acuity, and this is all the more so in those with PD. The fact is, Parkinson's can affect cognition, most often mildly but occasionally severely. Keeping your brain stimulated by reading, playing games, and doing puzzles and crosswords helps maintain your mental acuity. Social interactions with friends and family also are very helpful in this regard. There are many websites and apps available that provide stimulating games and puzzles.

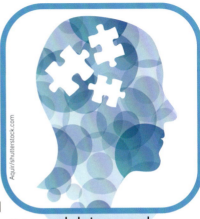

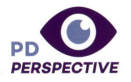

PD PERSPECTIVE

"It does not matter how slowly you go as long as you do not stop."
–Confucius

Life With **PARKINSON'S**

Me & My Parkinson's

 Is it safe (and legal) for me to continue driving?

Most states do not have specific guidelines regarding Parkinson's and driving. Yet, people with PD do develop slowed reaction times, problems with spatial judgment, and a reduced ability to process visual and spatial information. If a person with PD has a fender bender or tends to drive across traffic lanes or rush around corners, then they may have developed problems accurately judging distances.

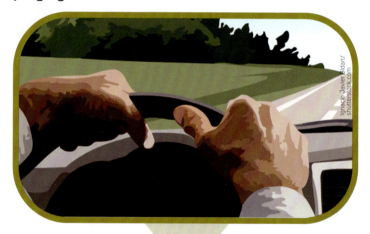

Some people with PD may have sleepy spells from medicine or insomnia, or even sleep attacks, and others may find it is difficult to move adequately behind the wheel. Continued driving is possible but needs to be assessed regularly in order to keep the person with Parkinson's, and anyone else, safe on the road. Although there is no motor vehicle requirement that says that someone with PD needs to stop driving, *what is required* **is to be able to safely drive**.

Frequently Asked Directions Along the Journey

It is important for those with Parkinson's to continually assess their ability to drive. At some point, a person with PD may realize on their own that the time has come to give up the convenience and luxury of driving. That realization may have been sparked by friends or family, who expressed concern, or by the professional opinion of a clinician or **driver rehabilitation specialist.**

About how long can I expect to continue to drive after my diagnosis?

Symptoms of PD and related abilities to drive are different for every individual with Parkinson's. Thus, people with Parkinson's should discuss their driving with their physicians at least once a year. If there are concerns, then a consultation with a driver rehabilitation specialist might be in order. These specialists will assess your driving and might recommend procedures or devices that will help your driving. The website for the Association for Driver Rehabilitation Specialists (aded.net) includes a member directory that is searchable by state.

Parkinson's medicines can sometimes cause drowsiness, confusion, dizziness, and even blurred vision, all of which can impair driving ability.

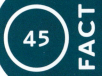

FACT 45

Life With **PARKINSON'S**

Me & My Parkinson's

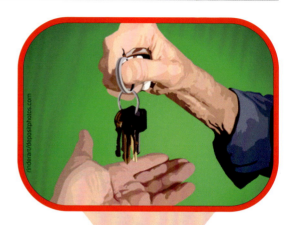

 I have been driving for 50 years! How can I possibly give up my keys?

 Giving up driving can be a difficult decision, but you should be content in the knowledge that for the safety of others, you have made the right choice. Remember that your family and friends, who make up your support network, will no doubt be available to help you with your transportation needs. And it doesn't hurt to remind yourself that driving can be stressful and cars can be financially taxing, whereas walking and biking will yield positive results.

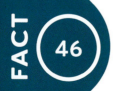

A person with Parkinson's can have his or her ability to drive assessed by a driver rehabilitation specialist.

Frequently Asked Directions Along the Journey

 We both recently retired, and we love to go on road trips to explore new places. Does my PD mean no more traveling?

 Absolutely not, *you can still travel!* Before each "big" trip it is always advisable to review your plans with your physician or other clinician. An important consideration is making sure you have enough medicines on hand for the entirety of the trip. Also, getting help traveling to and from the airport, and within the airport, should be prearranged. The **European Parkinson's Disease Association (EPDA)** (epda.eu.com) has a handy downloadable **Parkinson's Passport** that can hold information about the medicines you are taking, which you can take along with you when traveling.

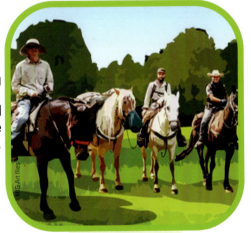

The medicine you bring along with you on your trip should be stored in the original bottles, and a bit more than needed should be included, since travel snafus can delay your return. You should continue to take your medicines following the same schedule as before. Use of a medical bracelet or wallet card to identify you as a person with PD is important in the event others need to know about your diagnosis.

Life With **PARKINSON'S**

 ## Me & My Parkinson's

Some additional PD-related travel tips

- Rest well before you travel and again upon arrival

- Don't overdo it! Rest is important, and eating and travel may take longer in an unfamiliar setting

- Locate and write down the location of the hospital and pharmacy nearest your destination(s). Identifying a physician familiar with Parkinson's disease near where you are traveling, and keeping their contact details with you, are also prudent precautions to take

- Your travel itinerary should allow plenty of opportunities for stops to use the toilet

- Make sure the facilities where you are going are acceptable for your needs, and check to make sure stairs can be avoided with either use of an elevator in the hotel or, failing that, book your room on the first floor

- If you are immobile or disabled, take a letter from your doctor stating that you are fit to travel and detailing your medicine. The Parkinson's Passport can help you explain your situation (find out more @parkinsonslife.eu)

- Deliberately hydrating the day before travel is a good idea to avoid trips to the bathroom on the day of travel. That said, keeping hydrated is important for a variety of health reasons and so should not be avoided

With proper preparation, people with Parkinson's can continue to enjoy travel and vacations.

Frequently Asked Directions Along the Journey

 Can I continue to drink alcohol?

Occasional alcohol consumption is usually fine as long as you don't have some other medical issue that prohibits it. The key is moderation, which might consist of a cocktail or a glass of beer or wine on a given day. However, this should be confirmed by your health care provider.

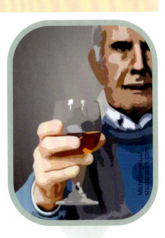

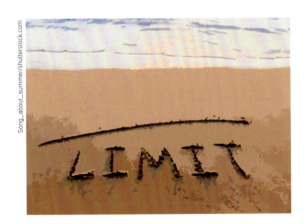

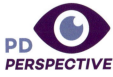

"Live each day; your disorder does not own you. Make every new day better; always remember, you are still in charge."
—Frank C. Church

Life With **PARKINSON'S**

 MILEPOSTS # Me & My Parkinson's

PD & My Job

How long can I keep working with Parkinson's?

Your work may be an important part of who you are, offering purpose, a social framework, and an income. For many people with PD, maintaining employment is vital for their ability to maintain their quality of life. The question of work typically comes up soon after receiving a PD diagnosis, and there is no set rule. Many people with Parkinson's can continue to work for years, and others can work but at a different job because they are not able to negotiate the physical demands of the original job. Still others can continue working with accommodations in place, such as different hours or workplace alterations.

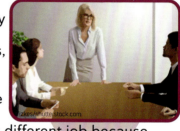

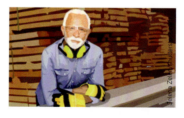

FACT 47

Disclosing to an employer that you have PD is the first step in setting up modifications or accommodations that may help you to continue doing your job well.

50 FACTS & MORE

Frequently Asked Directions Along the Journey

 How and when do I tell my employer about my Parkinson's diagnosis?

 Experts suggest holding off disclosing your PD diagnosis to your employer for a bit after you have received it, thus giving yourself time to adjust to the news and to learn as much as possible about the disease. It also will be helpful to get your physician's advice on how to approach your employer and the company.

> Don't wait especially long, however, as Parkinson's can have obvious and visible effects, such as tremor. You will want to make your employer and the **human resources (HR)** professional aware of your diagnosis so you can discuss time-off requirements and related workplace accommodations. You will need to have your employer and the human resources professional cognizant of your diagnosis so you can discuss time off requirements and workplace accommodations. Companies often have benefits or perks that may help, such as flexible work hours, **telecommuting**, or partial remote work. Your HR professional will be able to help you understand these. You should be ready to discuss these opportunities when you talk to your employer.

Your employer will likely be sympathetic when learning about your PD diagnosis. Still, their position requires that they be concerned about how it will affect getting the work finished on time.

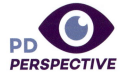
PD PERSPECTIVE

"Life is 10% what happens to me and 90% of how I react to it."
–Helen Keller

Life With **PARKINSON'S**

MILEPOSTS ## Me & My Parkinson's

 How is my PD discussion with my employer going to go? Any tips?

 On the next page is a sample list of talking points/positions offered as a conversation planning guide for addressing your first PD conversation with your employer.

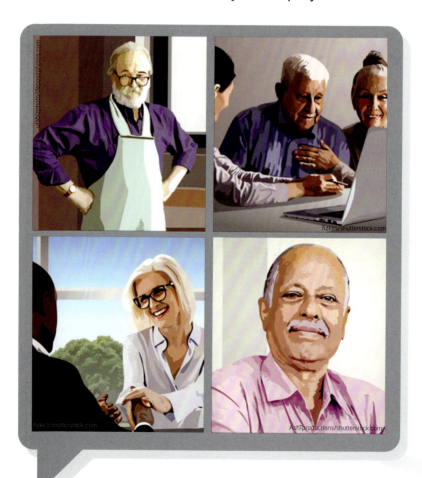

50 FACTS & MORE

Frequently Asked Directions Along the Journey

1 I've recently been diagnosed with Parkinson's disease, which is a fairly common disorder.

2 Thankfully, progression of the disease is usually pretty slow. There are medicines that help, and it is likely that I can continue working effectively for many years without significant problems. Eventually, it will affect my musculoskeletal coordination.

3 I need to tell you and human resources about the PD diagnosis so that I can use any available health benefits the company offers.

4 My physician has told me that it is likely I will be able to perform my job duties for several more years. I am personally very confident that this is so.

5 My physician suggested I may need some workplace accommodations in the future, but these are readily available and quite effective.

6 I know that this is not ideal but I'm sure that together we can implement solutions for my workplace that will allow me to continue to work hard for the company.

7 Thank you for this meeting and I appreciate your support.

Life With **PARKINSON'S**

 ## Me & My Parkinson's

 ### Should I tell my coworkers about my PD?

 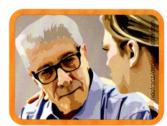 Telling fellow employees with whom you are close is advisable. Your closest coworkers will begin to notice symptoms at some point so letting them know about your diagnosis will give them the information they will need to understand what you are going through. Without that knowledge, rumors might pop up that are far from the truth.

Be open with them about Parkinson's, perhaps even offering them a printed overview of the disease so that they can learn more and rebut inappropriate comments by others. Make sure your fellow coworkers know that you will continue to do your job as effectively as you have in the past, and that you don't expect that to change anytime soon.

 ### What workplace rights are included in the Americans with Disabilities Act (ADA)?

 The ADA prohibits workplace discrimination based on disability, as long as the employee can continue to perform the job with reasonable accommodations. There are subtleties to this act, including the interpretation of what is reasonable. Also, smaller companies are not necessarily required to keep a person employed if the accommodations represent a substantial cost. So getting to know the details behind the ADA is an excellent idea. Your company's HR professional should be able to help you with this.

Frequently Asked Directions Along the Journey

 How do I apply for disability benefits?

 First, talk to your company's HR professional, or if the company has one, its benefits officer. Either person should be able to explain in detail the benefits that you may rightfully claim, both for you and your immediate family.

Details of disability benefits to understand

- Disability policies usually pay out a predefined percentage of your salary while you are disabled

- Pros and cons of early retirement

- Payment options from retirement accounts

- **Flexible spending accounts**, used to pay medical expenses not covered by insurance

- Medical insurance coverage of the costs for medicines

- Possibility of getting **long-term care insurance**, or using it if that is an option

- Possible benefits from various Social Security, **Medicare**, and **Medicaid** programs

 Flexible Spending Accounts can be used to pay insurance deductibles, or to pay medical or dental bills that are not covered by insurance.

Life With **PARKINSON'S**

Me & My Parkinson's

PD & My Finances

What about medical coverage and different types of insurance?

Knowledge of health insurance coverage and its relationship to employment is vital, yet complex. In some cases, employees may be able to continue to get the same health insurance if they stop working, until they qualify for Medicare or reach retirement age. In other cases, employers may limit continued insurance coverage for up to 18 months.

People with Parkinson's often get health insurance through Medicare,

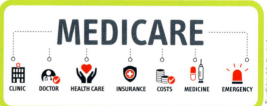

the federal government's health insurance program. To qualify for Medicare, you must be 65 years or older and be eligible for Social Security or Railroad Retirement benefits. Individuals who are younger than 65 years, must be eligible for disability benefits.

A person with PD, or their caregiver, should endeavor to become an expert in the world of insurance, including disability and long-term care insurance, either through their own research or discussions with others in their personal network.

Some insurance policies offer caregiving-related coverage for items such as **home health aides**, but often the costs may initially require payment by the individual.

50 FACTS & MORE

Frequently Asked Directions Along the Journey

 What are some key PD-related financial considerations to keep in mind?

 With this illness comes expenses, including those related to insurance, medicine, home modifications, and hiring of in-home helpers. As the disease progresses, individuals with PD may have to adjust their work schedule, or even stop working entirely. Costs may be incurred for services such as speech, occupational, or physiotherapy. There also may be additional unforeseen costs for nursing care or special therapeutic equipment.

A **financial plan** developed with the assistance of a financial planner is a wise step. Remember that a financial plan is not set in stone; revisiting it on a regular basis is advised.

Estate planning is also suggested so that you can appropriately provide for your loved ones after your death. Estate planning includes creation of a **will** and **advance directive**, and also designation of a **power of attorney** and **health care proxy**.

It is critical to think about and plan for the financial impact of your PD diagnosis as early as possible. It is important to find out whether you are eligible for any and all benefits that might help you recover from certain financial losses.

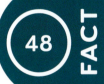

FACT 48

Life With **PARKINSON'S**

Me & My Parkinson's

What should I do about financial concerns as my Parkinson's progresses?

At some point, the complete details of your financial life need to be written down. Once that is done, this information needs to be periodically updated.

Organizing one's affairs sounds like a long and complicated chore, and in truth it can be, but the best way to do it is to start at a logical point and work from there. You may wish to start by creating a list of assets, which would include bank accounts, as well as insurance policies, stocks and bonds, contents of safe deposit boxes, and valuables like jewelry or antiques. This list should be updated at least annually and kept somewhere handy, likely together with your current will, **power of attorney**, and other important papers.

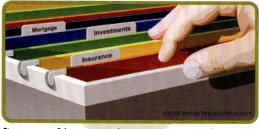

Originals should be stored in a secure place such as a safe, with the bank, at your lawyer's office, or in a fireproof box. Make sure you inform someone else where these important papers are stored. You may want to send a photocopy of the documents to another family member or close friend. One strategy that is sometimes suggested is to renew your will annually, so that any future argument about whether you were of sound mind is nullified.

Frequently Asked Directions Along the Journey

Ideally, financial planning should be addressed soon after the diagnosis of PD. As noted above, there are many concerns to consider, and these may change with age and severity of PD symptoms. Having a well-thought-out financial and estate plan will help both you and your family address the challenges of the disease, and keep related stresses at bay.

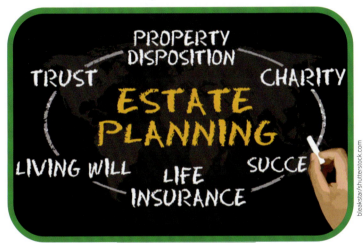

A lesser-known challenge is related to micrographia (page 28), the term for the tendency among people with Parkinson's to have handwriting that shrinks over time. This creates the unexpected challenge of safeguarding your right to use your signature, even as it evolves. Because of the changing nature of the signature, you may have to engage a lawyer to ensure that you will continue to be able to sign documents with authority.

Life With **PARKINSON'S**

 ## Me & My Parkinson's

Financial "To Do's" for people with Parkinson's

 • Convert to **electronic banking** if you haven't already; this will mean you can forego physical trips to the bank

 • Keep financial statements and legal documents well organized and continuously updated

 • Micrographia may alter your writing and penmanship, so make sure your bank has a recent sample of your signature

 • Payment with so-called Chip and PIN (personal identification number) credit and debit cards will allow you to only enter a few numbers on the keypad

 • Ensure that all passwords and PINs are stored somewhere safe. Make sure the passwords you use are not obvious or too simple, and don't use the same password for multiple sites. There are handy password programs available that create and store your passwords—stronger passwords that mix upper- and lowercase letters, numbers, and symbols—for you

 Financial planning information and tools are available from leading financial planners and disability consulting services, such as Allsup (allsup.com).

Frequently Asked Directions Along the Journey

 Are there any programs that offer financial assistance for people with PD?

 There are a few programs that might help with such things as the costs of medical equipment, home adjustments, and medicines.

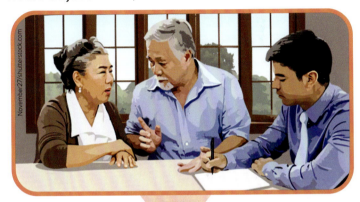

The Melvin Weinstein Parkinson's Foundation (MWPF; mwpf.org) is available for those who qualify. MWPF offers help for the purchase of medical equipment, such as wheelchairs, walkers, and canes, as well as other expenses, including home health care.

You also might find the nearest **Area Agency on Aging** office via the **Eldercare Locator Service** (eldercare.gov), which lists financial aid and other programs for seniors. Examples include programs like Meals-on-Wheels, Medicaid/Medicare, food stamps, low-income energy assistance programs, and advice on low-cost senior housing. There is also a list of pharmaceutical companies at **Parkinson.org** that lower costs of medicines for people with Parkinson's.

Life With **PARKINSON'S**

Me & My Parkinson's

An advance directive is a document that formalizes your demands for health care for such time when you might not be able to articulate them yourself. The neurologic effects of Parkinson's progress over time, and dementia may develop. An advance directive lets everyone on your health care team and your family know what you want done and not done under certain conditions. The directive should name a particular person or group of people who are authorized to speak and make decisions on your behalf. You should keep other important documents with the advance directive, including your latest medical and financial information, insurance documents, pertinent family documents (such as attorneys, accountants, clergy), and property documents, among others.

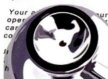

50 FACTS & MORE

Frequently Asked Directions Along the Journey

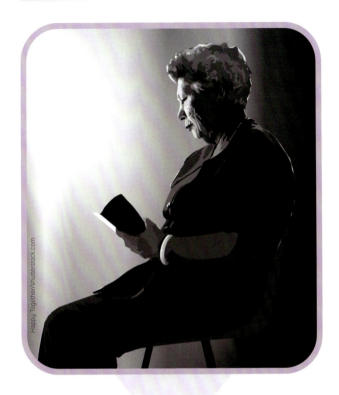

Financial planning and advance directives are best accomplished by considering the advice from multiple sources, and these very important documents should be periodically updated. It is never too early to consider preparing an advanced directive, but there may come a time when it is too late to offer significant input.

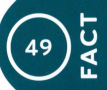

FACT 49

Partners & Caregivers

My partner has just been diagnosed with Parkinson's. What are the implications for me?

It's critical that caregivers and partners strive to increase their PD-related health literacy (page 42). Some couples will find that their relationship grows stronger when one of them has received a diagnosis of PD. Communicating openly and honestly is key. Relationships may change as symptoms change, but with good communication you can assist your partner as he or she adjusts to the evolving situation. You should strive to talk honestly with each other about any evolving problems in your relationship: what is and is not working. The Davis Phinney Foundation for Parkinson's has a self-assessment tool to help with relationships (davisphinneyfoundation.org).

> Facial masking, when the face of a person with PD is more rigid and slower to react (page 32), is a challenge for partners as expressions are important to communication. An unresponsive, blank facial demeanor, or a quiet voice, may be interpreted by others as a lack of interest, or worse. It will be important to remember this, and to educate others about it, so it will not adversely affect relationships.

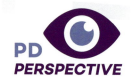

"It's not what we have in life but who we have in our life that matters."
–Maya Angelou

Frequently Asked Directions Along the Journey

What do I need to know about being a caregiver for someone with Parkinson's?

Being a caregiver is often a rewarding experience but can also be emotionally and physically straining, particularly if the caregiver is older. There might also be an economic disincentive as caregivers sometimes have to reduce or even give up their work hours. With these stresses come the possibility of a shifting relationship with the person with Parkinson's. Adjusting to these shifts will be a vital part of negotiating your caregiver role successfully.

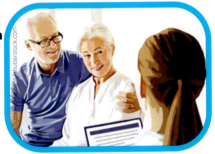

Caregivers should endeavor to remain positive. Positivity will no doubt not only help you but also the person with PD. Since the person you are taking care of will feel down from time to time, it is important to remember to actively try to boost their mood. This support is beneficial and should be mutual: The next time, the person with PD may well be boosting your mood.

Sometimes, people may feel that their caregiving role has taken over and that they are no longer seen as a spouse, partner, or loving family member. This feeling is not unusual and may need to be discussed so that it doesn't bring unnecessary tension into the relationship.

Life With **PARKINSON'S**

MILEPOSTS Partners & Caregivers

Being a PD caregiver is exhausting ... how do I safeguard my own well-being and identity?

First, be aware of your own needs and dedicate some time to yourself and no one else. The job of caregiving is a demanding one, so make sure you get the sleep you need, eat healthy, and take time to relax. It is perfectly understandable and natural to react with concern to new caregiver responsibilities, but remain vigilant for signs of depression, anxiety, unhappiness, prolonged fatigue, or resentment. **If you find yourself in emotional trouble, seek help from appropriate clinicians. Not attending to these feelings may worsen them or cause a crisis in your relationship with the person with PD**.

> It is an appropriate concern for clinicians looking after your partner with Parkinson's to learn that you as the caregiver are feeling overly stressed. If that's the case, feel free to speak up. As the caregiver, you are a vital part of the medical team that is helping the person with PD. If you can't help or you feel too stressed by helping, then intervention, possibly by getting assistance elsewhere, is called for.

For self-evaluation, you can access the **Caregiver Self-Assessment Questionnaire**, from the **American Medical Association** at healthinaging.org or use the **Parkinson's Foundation Caregiver Self-Assessment** at parkinson.org.

Frequently Asked Directions Along the Journey

Signs of caregiver-related emotional distress

• Irritability	• Trouble concentrating
• Anxiety	• Changes in appetite
• Lack of energy	• Substance abuse
• Overwhelming tiredness	• Loss of interest in things you normally would enjoy
• Mood swings	• Feeling too controlled
• Loss of emotional control	• Unusual physical symptoms
• Insomnia	• Thoughts of death or suicide

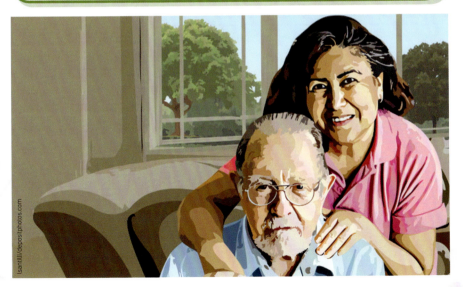

Life With **PARKINSON'S**

 Partners & Caregivers

Preparing for a Caregiver Role

 How can I best prepare myself for my caregiver role?

 Caregivers are an important part of the security net that should be built up to safeguard a person with PD. The role that the caregiver plays becomes ever more vital as the disease progresses. The caregiver role is an increasingly demanding one, and as such, caregivers need to learn to care not only for their Parkinson's charge but also for themselves.

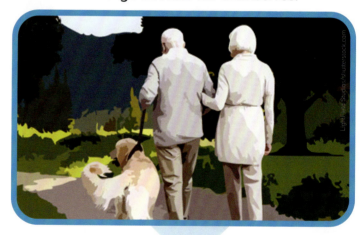

 There is a comprehensive caregiver's guide, Caring and Coping, available without charge online or by calling the **Parkinson's Foundation Helpline** (800-4PD-INFO [473-4636]).

Frequently Asked Directions Along the Journey

Important reminders for caregivers

- Perfection is not a real-life option. Show yourself compassion

- The caregiver should have scheduled break periods to decompress; you can't be on call all the time

- Caregiving can be an emotional experience, and all emotions are acceptable. A journal can sometimes be helpful to keep track and be aware of emotional changes

- Don't be afraid to call in outside help when the caregiving role becomes too much to handle

- Try to engage in enjoyable activities with the person with PD. Having fun is good for both of you

- Remember to safeguard your own health by maintaining a good diet, exercising, and getting a good night's rest

Caregivers should strengthen ties to family and friends, senior support groups, religious and civic institutions, and community organizations. There are excellent support groups for people who take care of those with PD such as **caring.com.**

Life With **PARKINSON'S**

Partners & Caregivers

Appointments & Insurance

 Should I attend the medical appointments?

Even if, in the beginning, the person with PD in your care is capable of getting themselves to their appointments, you should probably go along to ask questions, take notes, and share your unique perspective on symptoms or other issues that he or she may not bring up, such as sleeping problems or mood disorders. Keep a running list of questions to bring with you. It's also helpful to have a calendar (paper or digital, whatever works!) to keep track of physician and therapy appointments. You can also use a calendar to track medicines and keep notes about any side effects.

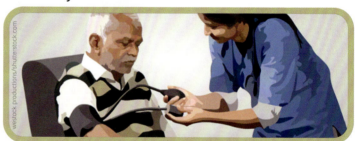

 All this insurance! How is this going to work?

If you were always the one who handled questions about insurance coverage, great; but if not, you may want to familiarize yourself with the terms of your health insurance. You'll need to know details about if and to what extent your plan covers prescriptions, therapy sessions, and other unexpected items.

Frequently Asked Directions Along the Journey

As a caregiver, you are in a unique position to note changes in symptoms, abilities, and moods. You are able to note new behaviors or abilities, especially after adjustments in medicine or therapy. Changes can appear in subtle ways that an individual with PD may not always immediately realize—for example, that he or she shouldn't drive anymore, or that there's a risk for falling or getting hurt. It can be hard to remind them of things they can't safely do. In these cases, consider asking a social worker or therapist for advice.

 I get so frustrated with the curveballs. How can I better handle the often abrupt changes to our plans?

Symptoms may vary over time and even from day to day. Try to be patient and flexible if, say, you had plans to do something that are now being derailed by a bad day. Try to give the person with Parkinson's in your care the best possible chance to do certain tasks independently before stepping in to assist them out of frustration.

Can you remove some tasks from either your own or his or her plate? For example, should you take over bill paying (if this task was their responsibility)? Or hire someone to do yard work? Talk to each other frequently in order to avoid miscommunication and resentment over changes you may propose.

Life With **PARKINSON'S**

Partners & Caregivers

PD Medicine Management

There are a lot of different medicines to manage with PD. What do I need to know about them?

Managing symptoms requires taking prescribed medicines at a specific dosage and at specific times (see "adherence" page 63). As the caregiver, you may have to oversee this. Forgetting to take medicine(s) may contribute to not being able to function as well as possible. To avoid making mistakes or having to bug or nag, develop a tool you both agree works, such as a smartphone reminder or a hard-to-miss wall calendar. Being consistent with medicine can make a big difference in both of your lives and lifestyles.

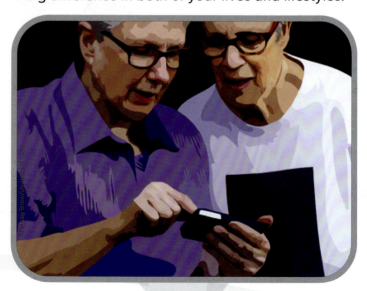

Frequently Asked Directions Along the Journey

PD medicine & caregivers

- Timing is crucial with Parkinson's medicine, as they must be taken on time, every time (page 63). An effective strategy is to set alarms on a smartphone–either yours or the person's with PD–for when to take the medicine. Another idea is to refill all pill boxes a week or more at a time. This has the dual benefit of getting all medicines ready beforehand, but also allows you to check the pill box to see if the pills have indeed been taken

- Medicines should always be stored in a safe place away from access by children and pets

- If pill swallowing issues develop, ask qualified care providers for advice

- It may be helpful to have a spare pill box filled appropriately with a couple days' worth of medicines (stored in a safe place) in case of hospitalization (where timely access to them may not always be possible)

- Financial support may be available for many PD medicines. Check online, with your pharmacy, or ask your health care provider for information

- Mail ordering Parkinson's medicines may be cost-effective; however, it may not always work smoothly as changes in dosages for one or more medicines may commonly have to be adjusted by a health care provider for any number of reasons. You may want to talk to a pharmacist or the prescribing physician about this issue when planning to order a specific PD medicine by mail

Partners & Caregivers

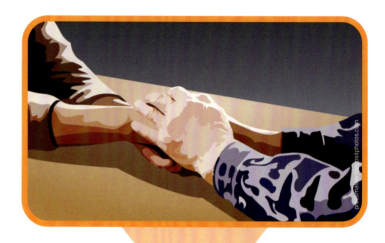

What changes in mental status can I expect in my spouse with Parkinson's?

As the disease of Parkinson's advances, changes in mental and motor capabilities will occur. As one's mental acuity and physical independence invariably diminish, the person with PD and the caregiver must adjust. Discussions that were once simple become less so, and in the end Parkinson's dementia may reduce or end constructive conversations. At these later stages, the person who was not only a caregiver but also a spouse or friend or family member may be increasingly defined solely by their caregiver role.

50 FACTS & MORE

Frequently Asked Directions Along the Journey

 What accommodations can I plan for and implement now in our home?

 As stated previously (page 123) falling is perhaps the most common and dangerous complication of PD. The good news is that by making certain adjustments and alterations, homes can be made much safer and more user-friendly for people with Parkinson's (page 184).

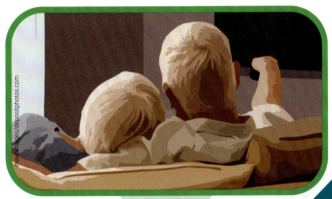

Making alterations to specific areas in one's home can significantly improve safety issues, as well as quality of life, for people with Parkinson's.

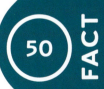

Life With **PARKINSON'S**

 Family, Friends, & Coworkers

How Can I Help?

 How can we help our parent with PD?

 Although day-to-day caregivers are critical members of the overall care team for people with Parkinson's, family members also play a vital role. They can be there to offer emotional support, physical assistance, and advice. Family members may take on personal care tasks like dressing, and may be supportive by doing household chores like cleaning, taking out the garbage, or paying bills.

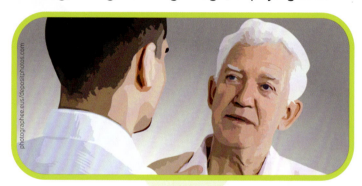

Family members should strive to increase their PD-related health literacy (page 42), be attuned to emotional changes, and be willing to step in when needed. Depression can affect the willingness of a person with Parkinson's to take care of themselves, but family members should intervene with a clinician when they see this developing as certain medicines and therapies can help. Family members should work to remind the person with PD of happy times and fun things from their family life in order to refocus their emotions on positive things.

Frequently Asked Directions Along the Journey

Communication Tips

 Do you have any tips to enhance communication with my best friend, and my neighbor, both of whom have Parkinson's?

 PD-related communication difficulties can affect family, friends, and caregivers. Communication problems can be frustrating to deal with and misunderstandings may arise.

Suggestions for communicating with a person who has Parkinson's

- Don't shout when speaking to them; talk normally

- Give a person with PD ample time to communicate

- Never sound impatient or stressed

- Listen carefully, and be in the same room where you can see each other

- Turn off any competing distractions such as music or a radio or television

- If you don't understand what they have said, ask them to repeat it a little louder and slower

- Don't interrupt, don't finish their sentences, and never walk away from them when their communication is slow

- Reassurance is helpful, and encouraging them to converse is good, but make sure they don't take that suggestion as pressure to talk

- Increasing PD-related health literacy can support understanding the potential causes of miscommunications

Life With **PARKINSON'S**

 Family, Friends, & Coworkers

Supporting Our Colleague With PD

 My colleague at work just shared a PD diagnosis; how can the company support their continued and valued contributions moving forward?

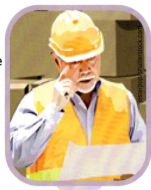

1. Work with your coworker in the creation of a plan for accommodations to workload. Break down large tasks into smaller and more manageable portions, and distribute work days and hours such that it allows for periods of rest.

2. Companies can provide educational opportunities/materials to increase PD-related health literacy (page 42). Open and honest dialogue among colleagues and the availability of PD educational materials in the workplace can help dispel misconceptions about Parkinson's and ease potential anxieties among staff. It's important to understand that misconceptions about PD are common, and that employers and coworkers can play a key role in educating others.

 Are there physical accommodations or technology we can implement at the office to assist our team member who has PD?

Explore different devices and software that could make working with their symptoms easier. There are many apps and technological accommodations that may alleviate stress in the workplace and help manage workloads and symptoms.

Frequently Asked Directions Along the Journey

The following organizations have missions dedicated to supporting people with Parkinson's, and/or their families and caregivers. You can search online for them by name, or locate their specific web addresses at the back of the book within the "Parkinson's Resources" section (page 211). This is just a sample listing. There are hundreds of organizations dedicated to Parkinson's-related support, so check online for more.

- **American Parkinson's Disease Association**
- **The Michael J. Fox Foundation**
- **Parkinson's Foundation**
- **The Davis Phinney Foundation for Parkinson's**
- **The Parkinson Alliance**
- **Parkinson's IQ + You**
- **Well Spouse Association (WSA)**
- **Caregiver Action Network (CAN)**
- **Family Caregiver Alliance (FCA)**

Life With **PARKINSON'S**

Keep on going while experiencing a better and healthier journey by following *Frank's Circle of Words**

FORTY-WINKS AND SLEEP SOME MORE

The brain is like a sponge that fills up all day with fluid; sleep allows the brain to drain, to renew, to fire-up strong upon waking; sleep is a very good thing.

FAITH

Believe in your ability to successfully navigate your life; trust in your loved ones to support your journey.

FULL-TIME

It takes time and effort to manage your life. You can find the time because managing your life well from this minute on will matter later in your life.

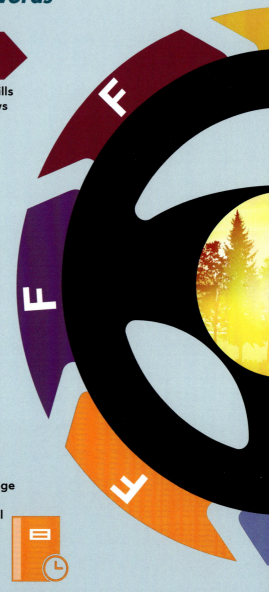

(Yes, they all begin with the letter "F"!)

FIT/FITNESS
Exercise as much as your body can take, then do some more. Getting/staying fit really matters in your battle with Parkinson's.

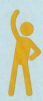

FORTITUDE
Stay strong in your effort with your adversity.

FOOD
Feed your brain properly, fuel your body well; it will make a difference.

FLEXIBLE (2 DEFINITIONS)
Stay flexible by stretching frequently; you've got a life-altering disorder, stay flexible and let your life follow what happens because it'll be okay.

*Adapted with permission from Frank C. Church.

Celebrities can use their status to speak candidly about their experiences living with Parkinson's. You may be surprised to learn how many well-known people, both past and present, not only learned to live successfully with Parkinson's, but also managed to create a platform to enhance broader social conversations about PD. These conversations help increase awareness and understanding of the condition, while personalizing Parkinson's for many with no other experience with it.

Alan Alda
Muhammad Ali
Sir Billy Connolly
Neil Diamond
Victoria Dillard
Michael J. Fox
Brian Grant

SECTION 4: THE FACES OF PARKINSON'S DISEASE

Jesse Jackson
Deborah Kerr
Ozzy Osbourne
David Parker
Davis Phinney
Janet Reno
Barbara Thompson

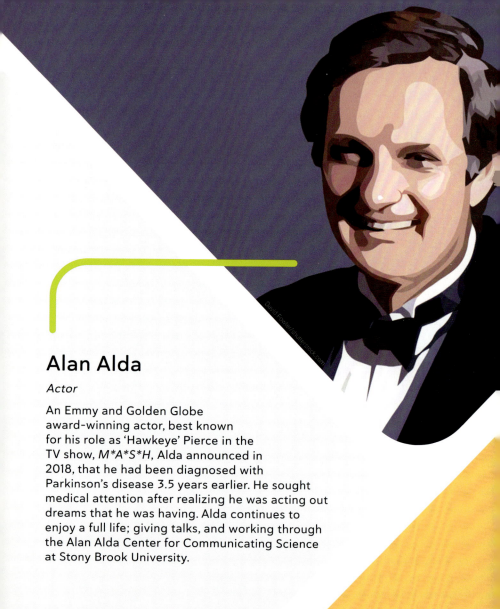

Alan Alda

Actor

An Emmy and Golden Globe award-winning actor, best known for his role as 'Hawkeye' Pierce in the TV show, *M*A*S*H*, Alda announced in 2018, that he had been diagnosed with Parkinson's disease 3.5 years earlier. He sought medical attention after realizing he was acting out dreams that he was having. Alda continues to enjoy a full life; giving talks, and working through the Alan Alda Center for Communicating Science at Stony Brook University.

Muhammad Ali

Professional boxer, activist, entertainer, and philanthropist

Although boxing fans began to notice a slowing of movement and speech during the 1970s, Ali was not diagnosed with Parkinson's disease until 1984, 3 years after retiring from boxing at the age of 42. Because he was such a public figure, researchers were able to study the early changes in his speech and movement in the years before his diagnosis, providing valuable insights into the early stages of his unique type of Parkinson's disease. After he retired from boxing, Ali remained active in philanthropic and activism activities, encouraging others to be as great as they can be.

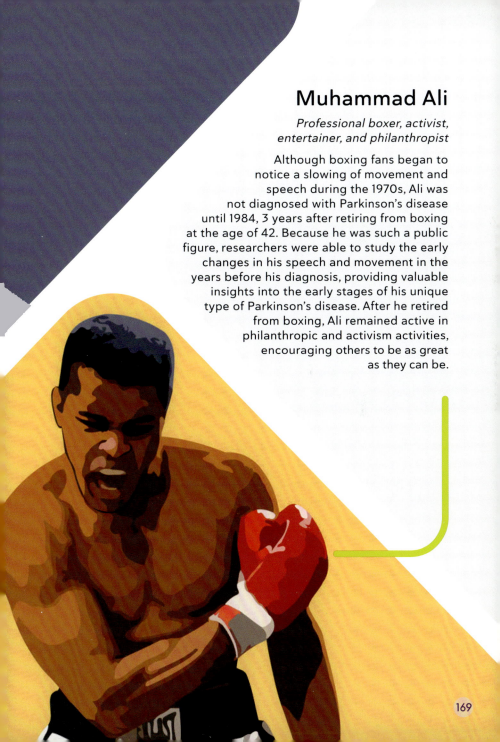

Sir Billy Connolly

Entertainer

A Scottish stand-up comedian and artist also known by his nickname 'The Big Yin' (the big one), Connolly revealed his diagnosis in 2013 and continued performing. He ended his tour activity in 2017 after finding that PD "made my brain work differently".

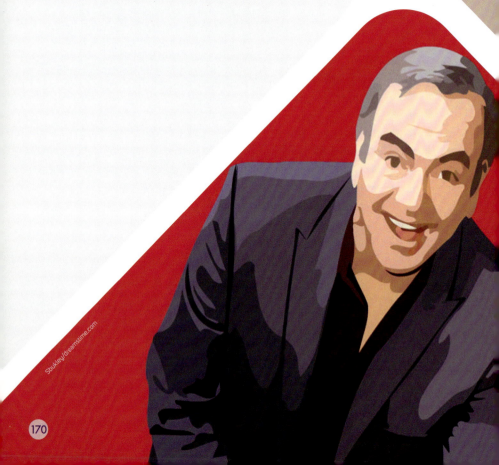

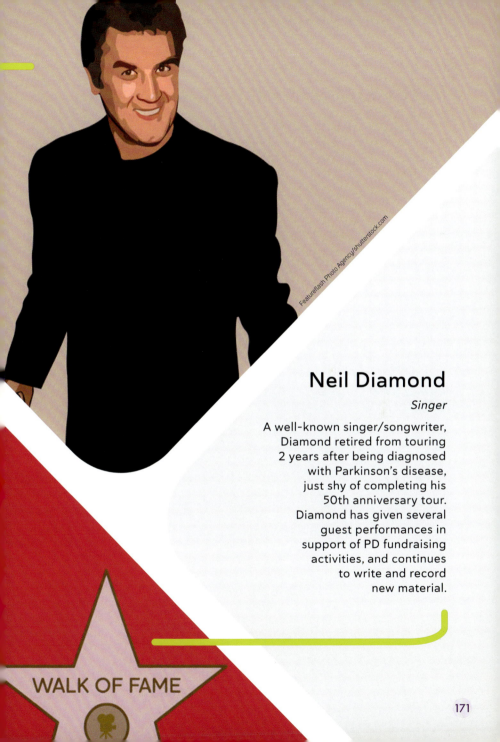

Neil Diamond

Singer

A well-known singer/songwriter, Diamond retired from touring 2 years after being diagnosed with Parkinson's disease, just shy of completing his 50th anniversary tour. Diamond has given several guest performances in support of PD fundraising activities, and continues to write and record new material.

WALK OF FAME

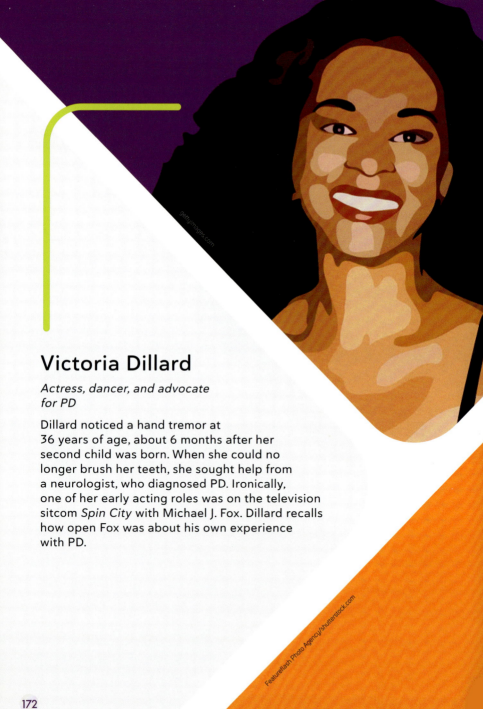

Victoria Dillard

Actress, dancer, and advocate for PD

Dillard noticed a hand tremor at 36 years of age, about 6 months after her second child was born. When she could no longer brush her teeth, she sought help from a neurologist, who diagnosed PD. Ironically, one of her early acting roles was on the television sitcom *Spin City* with Michael J. Fox. Dillard recalls how open Fox was about his own experience with PD.

Michael J. Fox

Actor

An American-Canadian actor best known for his roles in the sitcoms *Spin City* and *Family Ties*, and the *Back to the Future* movie series, Fox was 29 years old when he was diagnosed with early-onset Parkinson's disease in 1991. He retired from acting in 2000 because of his symptoms, and went on to establish The Michael J. Fox Foundation for Parkinson's Research (michaeljfox.org), which raises awareness about, and funds studies on Parkinson's disease.

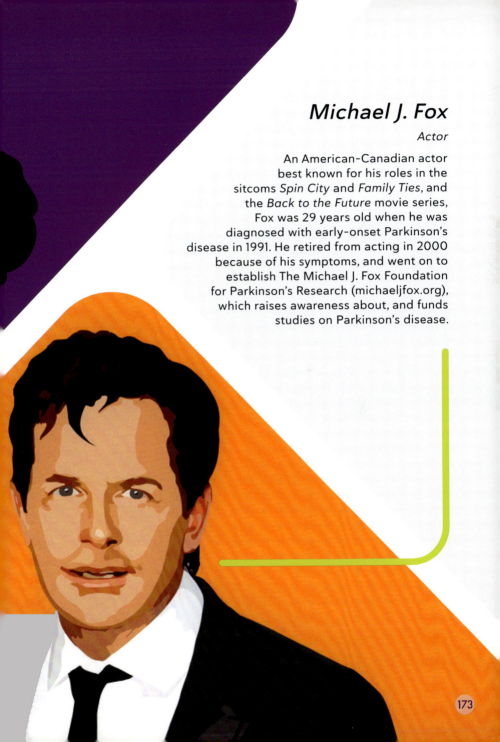

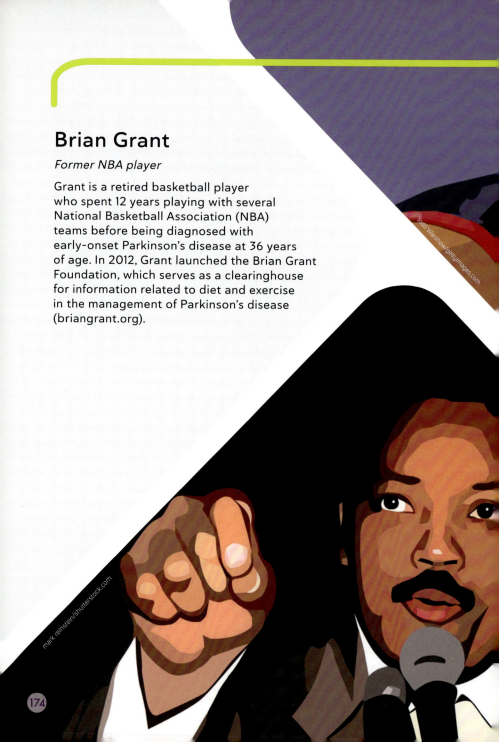

Brian Grant

Former NBA player

Grant is a retired basketball player who spent 12 years playing with several National Basketball Association (NBA) teams before being diagnosed with early-onset Parkinson's disease at 36 years of age. In 2012, Grant launched the Brian Grant Foundation, which serves as a clearinghouse for information related to diet and exercise in the management of Parkinson's disease (briangrant.org).

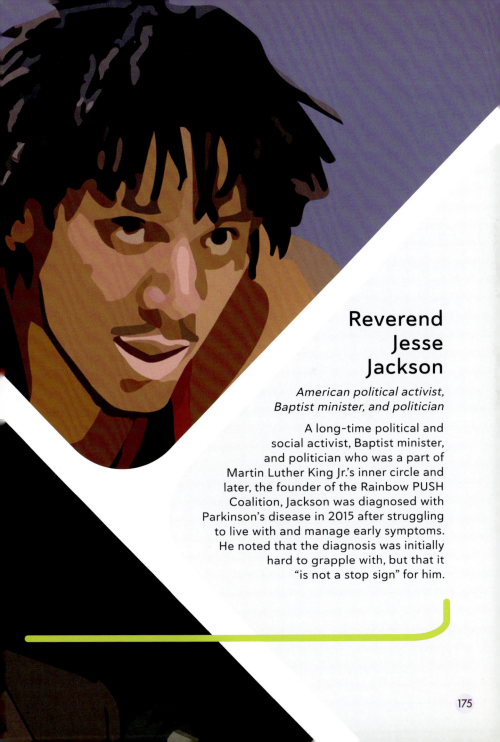

Reverend Jesse Jackson

American political activist, Baptist minister, and politician

A long-time political and social activist, Baptist minister, and politician who was a part of Martin Luther King Jr.'s inner circle and later, the founder of the Rainbow PUSH Coalition, Jackson was diagnosed with Parkinson's disease in 2015 after struggling to live with and manage early symptoms. He noted that the diagnosis was initially hard to grapple with, but that it "is not a stop sign" for him.

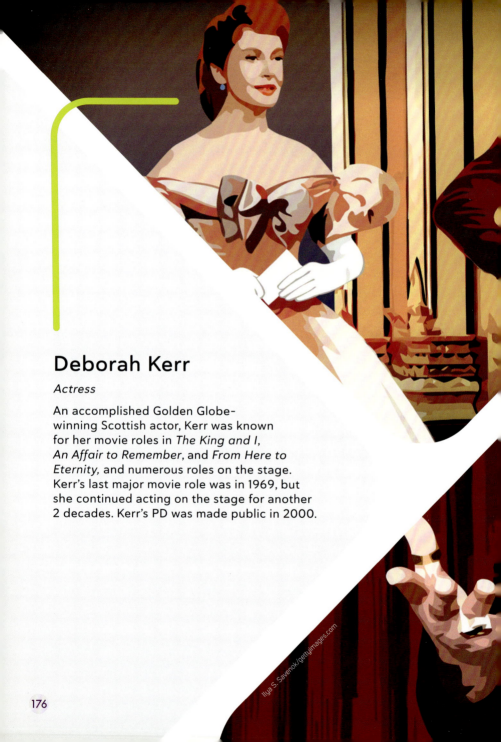

Deborah Kerr

Actress

An accomplished Golden Globe-winning Scottish actor, Kerr was known for her movie roles in *The King and I*, *An Affair to Remember*, and *From Here to Eternity*, and numerous roles on the stage. Kerr's last major movie role was in 1969, but she continued acting on the stage for another 2 decades. Kerr's PD was made public in 2000.

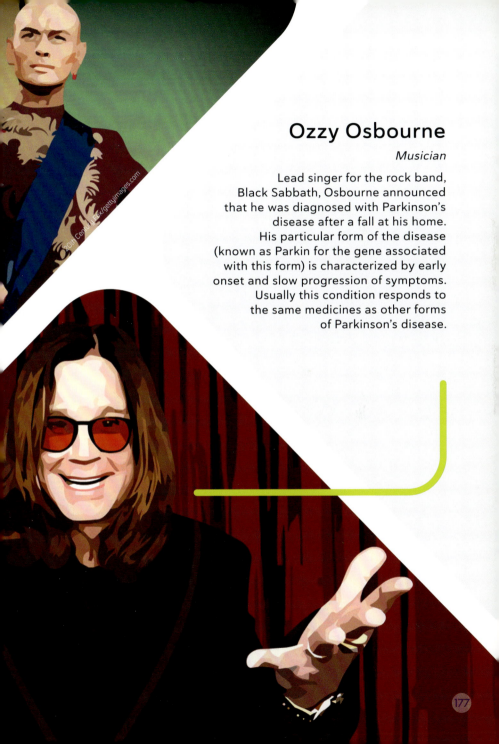

Ozzy Osbourne

Musician

Lead singer for the rock band, Black Sabbath, Osbourne announced that he was diagnosed with Parkinson's disease after a fall at his home. His particular form of the disease (known as Parkin for the gene associated with this form) is characterized by early onset and slow progression of symptoms. Usually this condition responds to the same medicines as other forms of Parkinson's disease.

David Parker

Former MLB player

Parker is a retired major league baseball player who played ball for 19 years with various clubs. Initially drafted by the Pirates in 1970, he moved to major league play in the 1973-74 season. In 2012, Parker was diagnosed with PD after a physician noticed his hand trembling and mentioned that he might have "a little touch of Parkinson's." Parker and his wife set up the DavidParker39 Foundation which supports awareness and research into PD (daveparker39foundation.com).

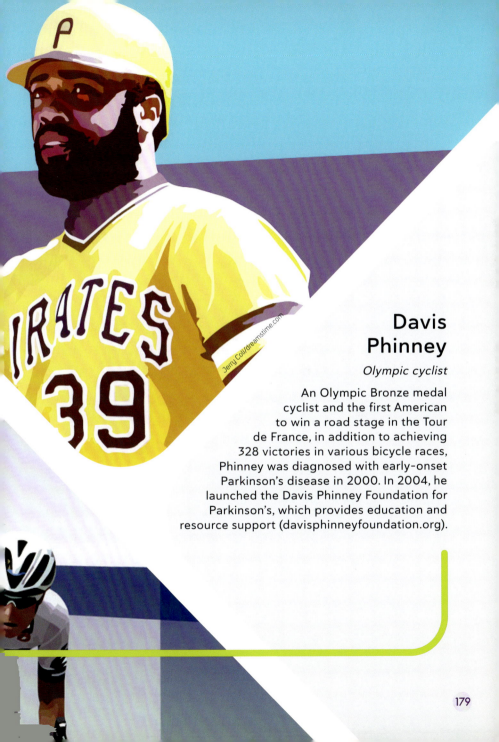

Davis Phinney

Olympic cyclist

An Olympic Bronze medal cyclist and the first American to win a road stage in the Tour de France, in addition to achieving 328 victories in various bicycle races, Phinney was diagnosed with early-onset Parkinson's disease in 2000. In 2004, he launched the Davis Phinney Foundation for Parkinson's, which provides education and resource support (davisphinneyfoundation.org).

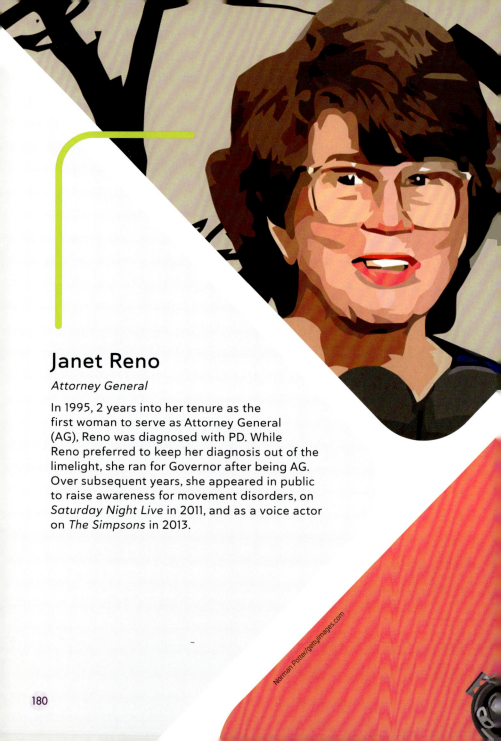

Janet Reno

Attorney General

In 1995, 2 years into her tenure as the first woman to serve as Attorney General (AG), Reno was diagnosed with PD. While Reno preferred to keep her diagnosis out of the limelight, she ran for Governor after being AG. Over subsequent years, she appeared in public to raise awareness for movement disorders, on *Saturday Night Live* in 2011, and as a voice actor on *The Simpsons* in 2013.

Norman Potter/gettyimages.com

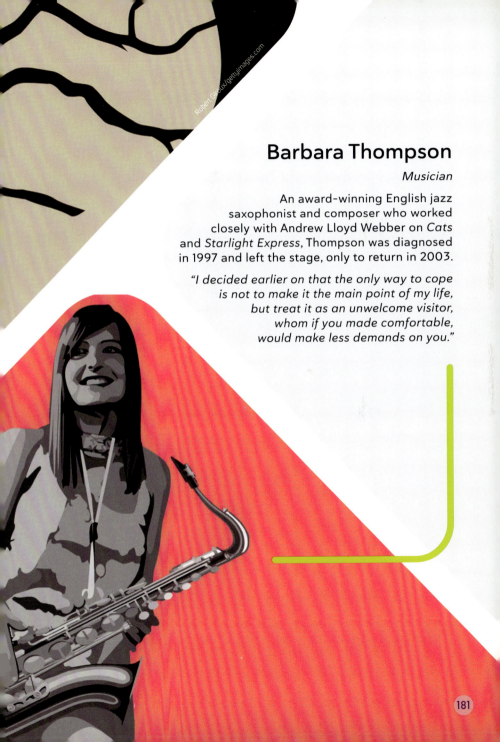

Barbara Thompson

Musician

An award-winning English jazz saxophonist and composer who worked closely with Andrew Lloyd Webber on *Cats* and *Starlight Express*, Thompson was diagnosed in 1997 and left the stage, only to return in 2003.

"I decided earlier on that the only way to cope is not to make it the main point of my life, but treat it as an unwelcome visitor, whom if you made comfortable, would make less demands on you."

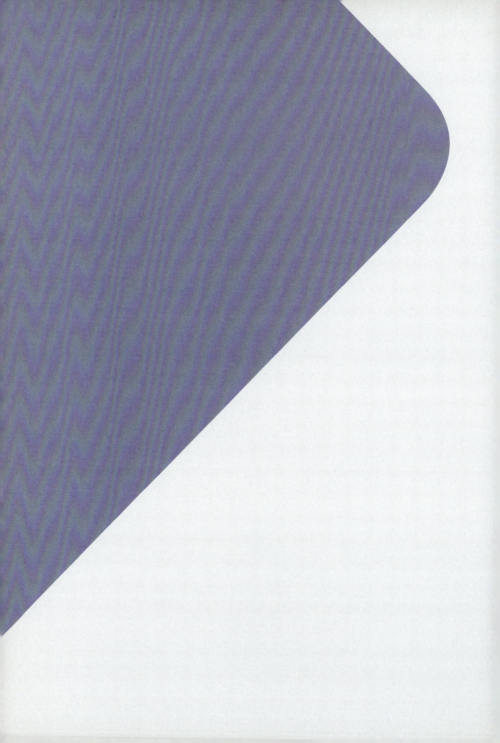

APPENDICES

APPENDIX A. PD Safety & Ease of Use

As discussed on page 31, falling is perhaps the most common and dangerous complication of PD because it can lead to fractures or head injuries. Additionally, because you are in your home more than any other place, it just makes sense to ensure that it is as safe and "PD user-friendly" as possible.

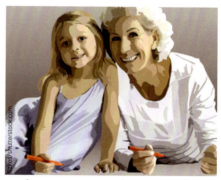

Being a person with PD means that there are certain strategies you can employ to make things as safe and functional as possible. Below are some tips for increasing safety in the home as well as general suggestions to think about regarding making life in the home a bit easier on the person with Parkinson's when dressing, eating, and moving about.

Flooring accommodations

Due to their unsteady gate at times, people with Parkinson's are prone to falls. Changes to flooring and floor coverings may help to prevent falls in the home. These adjustments can include:

Removing throw/area rugs

Avoiding trip zones, which are abrupt changes between types of surfaces (for example, carpet to tile)

Wide walking paths that allow easy access for people using walkers or wheelchairs

Having patterns in tiles or rugs that can be followed while walking

Removing clutter

Using non-skid surfaces

Changes for the Home

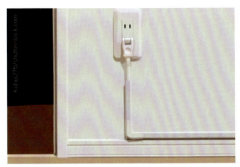

Bright lighting, both on flat surfaces and on stairs, can prevent confusion caused by shadows or glare. Use of light paint colors can also help visually. Night lights throughout the house are advised, including between the bedroom and bathroom. Furniture should be out of the way of frequently travelled pathways. Consider moving furniture so that there is a touch path that can be followed. All furniture should be situated so that it will not be tripped on or require the person with PD to turn to maneuver around. Furniture should be sturdy, non-rotating, and securely placed. Tape can be used to mark the ground to highlight foot placement at more difficult spots such as doorways or around corners, or next to the toilet.

did you know

Stairs should have sturdy railings and non-slip surfaces. For outdoor access, ramps can be built over exterior stairs. It is important to make sure these alterations are in accordance with local building codes.

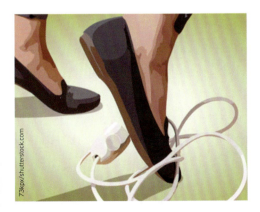

Cords from appliances or electronic devices should be secured and out of the way. Grab bars can be placed throughout the home in places where falls may be more likely. Stairs can be made more secure by adding handrails on both sides and using a non-skid surface.

APPENDIX A. PD Safety & Ease of Use

Additional changes

Other PD-related changes in the home may make life easier. For example, people with Parkinson's often find that lever-style door handles (vs knobs) are easier to use, while faucets and lamps that simply respond by touch are also key adjustments. Placing electrical outlets and power strips at a level higher than the floor can prevent the need to bend over, which reduces the risk for a fall.

Bedroom accommodations

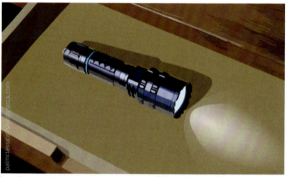

Making a few changes can help people with PD stay safe while getting in and out of bed. The bed's height should be adjusted so that feet can easily touch the floor when sitting on the edge. A grab bar or rope placed above the bed can make it easier to get out of bed, and some recommend using a bottom bed sheet made of a more slippery material than standard cotton or cotton mix. Using fewer layers on the bed (for example, not using a top sheet) can prevent getting tangled up. Keep items that might be needed during the night or in the morning, including a bottle of water, flashlight, and phone, near the bed. In addition, nighttime trips to the bathroom can be avoided by using a bedside commode.

Use of colored tape at the top and bottom of stairs or on each step helps people with PD who have a tendency to freeze (pages 30-31) while walking or have problems with depth perception.

Changes for the Home

You may find that certain types of clothing make walking and other movements safer and more comfortable. For instance, non-skid socks and lightweight shoes with Velcro or elastic laces may help prevent tripping or falls. Adaptive clothing such as those that use Velcro fasteners may make dressing easier than clothes with zippers or buttons.

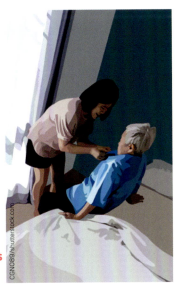

Dressing accommodations

Getting dressed can sometimes be a complicated and difficult task with PD, but it can be made easier with some changes.

> **Give yourself plenty of time to avoid last-minute rushing**
>
> **Do stretches beforehand and try to dress when symptoms are less pronounced**
>
> It may be easiest to dress while sitting on a chair that has arms. Avoid dressing while sitting on the bed, where you can easily slip off
>
> **Clothes should be hung on easily reached rods or stored in drawers that can be opened without bending down**
>
> A footstool or long-handled shoehorn can help with putting on shoes and socks

APPENDIX A. PD Safety & Ease of Use

A non-skid rubber bathmat in the bathtub or shower will help prevent slipping. Bathing can be made easier by using a handheld showerhead, or replacing a "climb-in" tub with a "walk-in" type. Use a liquid soap dispenser instead of bar soap, and a chest-height shelf to store commonly used items. Upgrade to powered versions of grooming tools instead of manual (razors, toothbrush, water flosser, etc).

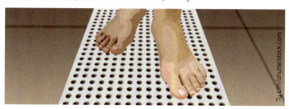

Bathroom and grooming accommodations

The bathroom is the room in your house that has the highest risk for falls and fall-related injuries. As such, there are many safety precautions you should take. Slippery tiles, wet surfaces, getting in and out of the tub, getting on and off the toilet, and the need to stand for long periods of time while washing hands, brushing teeth, or shaving can all make falls more likely.
Make the bathroom safer by:

- Putting grab bars near the toilet, tub, and shower
- Using a higher toilet seat with arm rests or a nearby grab bar
- Using a bench with a back rest in the shower
- Keeping floors clear or using rubber-backed bathroom rugs
- Sitting while shaving or brushing your teeth

Changes for the Home

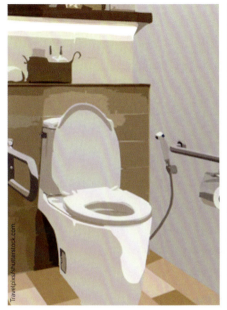 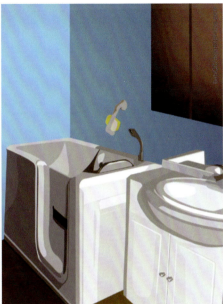

As shown above, increasing bathroom safety includes the appropriate addition of rails and handles, installing a walk-in tub, or a shower chair with a handheld shower head, and adjusting the heights of shelves commonly used.

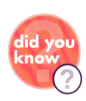

Going to the bathroom on a schedule can help to prevent falls. It may be helpful to limit fluid intake during the evening hours, avoid caffeine, and use a mild stool softener to make bowel movements more regular or predictable, if needed. These strategies may help prevent rushing to the bathroom or needing to take frequent trips to the bathroom at night.

APPENDIX A. PD Safety & Ease of Use

Kitchen and eating accommodations

Kitchen safety may be especially challenging for people with PD. Carrying heavy dishes, moving between the kitchen and dining room table, and reaching up to shelves can all cause problems. To be safe in the kitchen, consider using cabinet handles rather than knobs and store commonly used items nearby. If cutting or mixing is needed, tools with non-slip rubber bottoms (such as cutting boards and mixing bowls) or adaptive tools (such as knives) can prevent accidents.

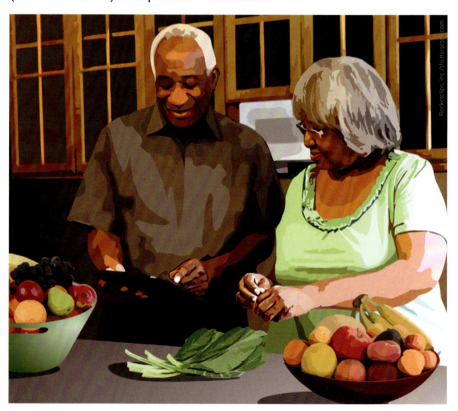

Changes for the Home

An occupational therapist can provide ideas that will help mitigate specific eating and dining challenges. Some ideas for changes include building handles on eating utensils or other tools so that they are easier to hold, placing non-slip materials under plates and bowls, and using a plate guard to help get food onto utensils.

The best foods for people with Parkinson's are those that can be cut into bite-size pieces and softer foods that are easier to chew and swallow. Food choices may need to be adjusted over time to ensure that you can continue to serve yourself. Using a napkin or apron to protect clothing will prevent the need to change clothes if spills occur. Mealtimes are a convenient time to have a beverage since you should drink 6 to 8 glasses of fluid per day (48 to 64 ounces per day).

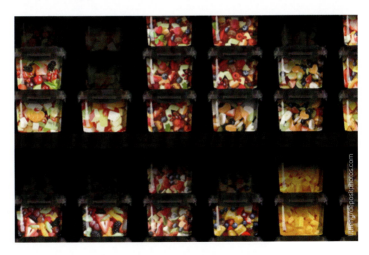

Buying pre-cut and pre-washed foods requires less use of sharp knives, which can be risky, and will reduce food preparation time in the kitchen.

Life With **PARKINSON'S**

APPENDIX A.   PD Safety & Ease of Use

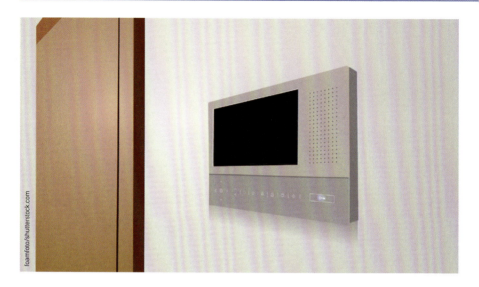

did you know?

Living alone can make some things about PD more challenging; however, some additional changes around the house and a good support system can help individuals live alone safely. For instance, installing a doorbell with a camera view can give you more control over when to open the door. Give a set of house keys and emergency phone numbers to a few trusted people with specific instructions about when they should be used. Consider use of a wearable alarm button to easily call for help if needed. Maintain a list of contact information for your support network and community services so that you can easily call someone when needed.

Changes for the Home

Mobility accommodations

Many people with PD continue to have good mobility for a long time. But, as symptoms change, some may need more support to get around. Your doctor or physical therapist can advise you about support tools such as a cane, walker, or wheelchair. Straight canes (those without extra feet at the base) and a rubber tip are the safest for people with PD. Hiking sticks or poles may be a better choice for people who want to maintain their posture while walking.

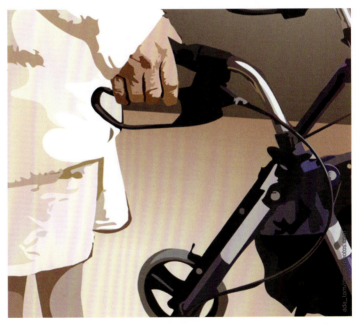

The safest walkers for people with PD have hand brakes and 4 or more large wheels that can swivel. Other helpful walker features may include a built-in seat, a basket to carry items, and even a laser. There are many types of wheelchairs available, each designed to address different needs.

APPENDIX B.   PD Abbreviations & Acronyms

ADLs: Activities of daily living
ADA: American's With Disabilities Act
AMA: American Medical Association
ANS: Autonomic nervous system
C/L: Carbidopa/Levodopa
CAN: Caregiver Action Network
CDS: Continuous dopaminergic stimulation
COMT: Catechol-O-methyltransferase
CNS: Central nervous system
DA: Dopamine agonist
DAWS: Dopamine agonist withdrawal syndrome
DBS: Deep brain stimulation
EDS: Excessive daytime sleepiness
EPDA: European Parkinson's Disease Association
ER: Extended-release
ET: Essential tremor
FADs: Frequently asked directions
FCA: Family Caregiver Alliance
fMRI: Functional magnetic resonance imaging
FOG: Freezing of gait
GDS: Geriatric depression scale
GP: General practitioner
HR: Human resources
HWP: Husband with Parkinson's
ICD: Impulse control disorder
ITT: Intention to treat
JPD: Juvenile Parkinson's disease
LCIG: Levodopa/carbidopa intestinal gel
L-dopa: Levodopa
LID: Levodopa-induced dyskinesia
MAO: Monoamine oxidase
MAO-B: Monoamine oxidase type B
MCI: Mild cognitive impairment
MDS: Movement Disorder Society

MDS: Movement disorder specialist
MDT: Multidisciplinary team
MDwP: Doctor with Parkinson's
MMSE: Mini Mental State Examination
MRI: Magnetic resonance imaging
MSA: Multiple system atrophy
MSA-P: Multiple system atrophy with Parkinson's symptoms
MWPF: Melvin Weinstein Parkinson's Foundation
ND: Neurodegenerative disease
NOH: Neurogenic orthostatic hypotension
OT: Occupational therapist
PBA: Pseudobulbar affect
PCA: Parkinson's care assistant
PCRN: Primary Care Research Network
PD: Parkinson's disease
PDD: Parkinson's disease dementia
PDP: Parkinson's disease psychosis
PET: Positron emission tomography
PNS: Parkinson's nurse specialist
PSW: Parkinson Support & Wellness
PT: Physiotherapist
PWP: Person with Parkinson's
RCT: Randomized controlled trial
RNA: Ribonucleic acid
RLS: Restless legs syndrome
SD: Standard deviation
SLT: Speech and language therapist
SPIRiTT: Specialist Parkinson's Integrated Rehabilitation Team Trial
SwP: Single with Parkinson's
TRAP: Tremor, rigidity, akinesia, postural instability
UPDRS: Unified Parkinson's Disease Rating Scale
WSA: Well Spouse Association
WWP: Wife with Parkinson's
YOPD: Young-onset Parkinson's disease

APPENDIX C. Glossary & Index

Numbers within brackets indicate page locations of glossary terms.

Acetylcholine (ACh): A neurotransmitter that can affect motor symptoms when levels increase and are not in balance with the dopamine levels [45, 71, 76]

Activities of daily living (ADLs): Routine tasks that can be performed without assistance by healthy people; difficulties experienced while performing these tasks can result in a reduced quality of life [122, 194]

Adenosine A_{2a} antagonists: Type of medicine used to treat Parkinson's disease that blocks adenosine in the brain to reduce "off" episodes resulting from long-term treatment with levodopa. This medicine is used as an add-on treatment to carbidopa/levodopa [70]

Adherence: The practice of taking a medicine as directed [63, 156]

Advance directive: A document (living will or power of attorney) that outlines how to address a person's medical decisions in the event that the person is unable to make those decisions [141, 146, 147]

Aggravators: Risk factors that aggravate the disease process and enable it to cause further damage and spread through the brain [20, 21]

Amantadine: A medicine that improves the symptoms of Parkinson's disease. Amantadine has been shown to decrease peak-dose dyskinesia in people with Parkinson's disease without worsening other symptoms [70, 71]

American Medical Association (AMA): The largest organization of physicians in the United States (ama-assn.org) [150, 194]

American Parkinson's Disease Association: The largest grassroots organization committed to fighting Parkinson's disease through education, support, and research (apdaparkinson.org) [163]

Americans With Disabilities Act (ADA): An act that prohibits workplace discrimination based on disability as long as the employee can continue to perform the job with reasonable accommodations [138]

Amino acid: A basic substance in the body that serves as a building block for proteins, as well as certain neurotransmitters [47, 48]

Anosmia: The loss of the sense of smell [26]

PD Keywords & Definitions

Anticholinergic: Medicine that blocks the effect of acetylcholine and helps control tremors; however, there are many side effects [71]

Antioxidants: Substances that prevent oxidation, which potentially can damage cells of organisms [37]

Anxiety: A common non-motor symptom experienced by people with Parkinson's disease [10, 29, 32, 60, 80, 81, 110, 150,151]

Apomorphine: A short-acting dopamine agonist used to treat "off" episodes of Parkinson's disease that may not be sufficiently controlled by increasing the frequency or amount of levodopa [64, 72]

Atrophy: The decrease in size of tissue or an organ caused by cellular shrinkage [27]

Autonomic functions: Involuntary body functions, such as breathing and swallowing [33, 98]

Autonomic nervous system: The complex system of nerves that controls the "automatic" activity of some of the internal organs, such as breathing, heartbeat, swallowing, or movement of the intestinal tract [126, 194]

Blood-brain barrier: A highly selective semipermeable border of endothelial cells that allows vital nutrients to reach the brain, while protecting the brain from unwanted substances [47, 48, 53, 64,65]

Bradykinesia: Slowness of movement; a major symptom of Parkinson's disease [23, 33, 74, 99]

Carbidopa: A medicine given in combination with levodopa for Parkinson's disease to improve the effectiveness and reduce side effects of levodopa; it prevents the body from using levodopa before it reaches the brain [56, 57, 58, 61, 64, 65, 70, 72, 73, 194]

Caregiver Action Network: A family caregiver organization dedicated to improving the quality of life of individuals caring for family members with chronic conditions or disabilities (caregiveraction.org) [163, 194, 211]

Caregiver Self-Assessment Questionnaire: Developed by the AMA, this questionnaire assesses a caregiver's stress and burden as a result of caring for a loved one [150]

APPENDIX C. Glossary & Index

Caring.com: A website that provides information and support for caregivers [153]

Catechol-O-methyltransferase (COMT): A special enzyme that breaks down dopamine and levodopa, thereby helping to regulate the amount of dopamine available to neurons in the substantia nigra [49, 51, 68, 194]

Catechol-O-methyltransferase inhibitor (COMT inhibitor): A type of medicine that may be used, along with carbidopa/levodopa therapy, in the treatment of symptoms of Parkinson's disease. COMT inhibitors block the action of the COMT enzyme [66, 68, 69, 70]

Center of Excellence Network: The Parkinson's Foundation's network of widely recognized medical centers that have specialized teams of knowledgeable clinicians that are up to date on the research, treatment, management of Parkinson's disease [52]

Central nervous system (CNS): The brain and spinal cord [92, 194]

Clinical trials: Experiments conducted in clinical research to evaluate an intervention, such as a medicine or a surgical procedure [2, 16, 21, 121]

Cognitive function: Mental abilities that process and understand knowledge (for example, learning and remembering) [73, 74]

Constipation: An alteration in stool frequency, consistency, and/or passage of stool. Parkinson's disease affects muscles and nerves in the gastrointestinal tract, slowing down the time it takes for the stomach to empty and for material to move through the intestines [26, 33, 94]

DaTscan: A special test that takes pictures of the brain to measure dopamine-containing neurons involved in controlling movement [27]

Davis Phinney Foundation for Parkinson's: A nonprofit organization committed to helping individuals with Parkinson's disease live well (davisphinneyfoundation.org) [38, 111, 148, 163, 179, 211]

Deep brain stimulation (DBS): A surgical procedure for the treatment of Parkinson's disease that involves the placement of wires (electrodes) into a specific area of the brain along with an impulse-generating battery under the collarbone. Symptoms related to

PD Keywords & Definitions

Parkinson's disease improve with the delivery of electric impulses to the brain [72, 73, 74, 84, 122, 194]

Delusions: Irrational beliefs that are not based on reality and resist any evidence to the contrary [29, 82]

Depression: A non-motor system that nearly half of people with Parkinson's may experience at some time in the course of their disease journey [3, 10, 26, 29, 32, 35, 73, 76, 78, 79, 80, 81, 92, 100, 150, 160]

Device-aided Parkinson therapies: Types of Parkinson's treatment options that involve the use of medical devices as well as surgical options (for example, levodopa/carbidopa intestinal gel infusion) [72]

Dietitian: An expert on diet and nutrition [119]

Diphasic dyskinesia: A type of dyskinesia that tends to affect the pelvis and legs, and occurs around the time the medicine levels in the blood are declining [62]

Dopamine: A chemical produced by the brain that helps send messages from one nerve cell to another. Individuals with Parkinson's have decreased amounts of dopamine in the substantia nigra, located deep in the brain. Dopamine in the substantia nigra coordinates the actions of movement, balance, and walking
[several mentions, see table of contents]

Dopamine agonist (DA): A medicine that can activate the dopamine receptors the same way that dopamine does [30, 64, 65, 70, 100, 101, 194]

Dopamine receptor: A receptor in the brain that receives dopamine and then generates an electric impulse in the next nerve cell to continue signal transmission along the chain of neurons that connect the brain and spine to individual muscles to create movement [45, 46, 48, 49, 64, 65]

Dream enactment behaviors: A sleep disorder in which a person has vivid, unpleasant dreams with vocal sounds and sudden and potentially violent arm and leg movements [26]

Driver rehabilitation specialist: A professional who assesses an individual's driving and recommends procedures or devices to provide solutions for people with disabilities [129, 130]

APPENDIX C.   Glossary & Index

Droxidopa: A synthetic amino acid precursor used to treat symptoms associated with neurogenic orthostatic hypotension, such as lightheadedness [88, 89]

Drug-induced parkinsonism: Parkinson's symptoms that have been caused by drugs used to treat other conditions [27]

Dyskinesia: Uncontrolled, involuntary movement that may occur in some people with Parkinson's disease and may be related to their long-term levodopa use and longer time with Parkinson's [49, 60, 62, 64, 70, 71, 72, 73, 74]

Dysphagia: Difficulty swallowing [33]

Dystonia: Uncontrolled muscle contractions in the legs, arms, neck, eyes, or trunk that are associated with Parkinson's disease [24, 34]

Early-onset Parkinson's disease: Diagnosis of Parkinson's disease before age 50; also known as young-onset Parkinson's disease [18, 173, 174, 179]

Electronic banking: Bank activity that can be performed 24 hours a day using a computer, ATM, debit card, or over the phone [144]

Enlarged prostate: Age-related condition in which the gland gets bigger; common among men over age 50 [95]

Entacapone: A COMT inhibitor used to treat Parkinson's disease [68]

Environmental toxins: Poisonous substances found in the environment such as in the air or water [17]

Enzymes: Proteins that act as a catalyst to accelerate a chemical reaction [49, 51, 56]

Essential tremor: A condition characterized by tremor in certain parts of the body, such as hands and head; may be mistaken for a symptom of Parkinson's disease [27, 194]

Estate planning: The process of planning the management and distribution of a person's estate in the event the person is incapacitated or dies [141, 143]

PD Keywords & Definitions

European Parkinson's Disease Association (EPDA): A European Parkinson's organization dedicated to providing advocacy, awareness, and support (epda.eu.com) [131, 194, 211]

Excessive daytime sleepiness (EDS): The inability to maintain wakefulness or alertness during the day, often due to lack of proper sleep at night [32, 90, 194]

Executive function: Describes a group of mental processes and cognitive abilities (working memory, reasoning) that influence goal-directed processes (organization, managing time, reasoning) [77]

Extended-release (ER): A long-acting version of a medicine [60, 70, 194]

Facial masking: Reduced facial expression; also known as hypomimia, sometimes simply called masking [32, 148]

Facilitators: Risk factors of Parkinson's disease that enable triggers to cause damage [20, 21]

Family Caregiver Alliance (FCA): A national nonprofit caregiver support organization committed to improving the quality of life of caregivers (caregiver.org) [163, 194, 211]

Financial plan: A plan that accounts for the income and expenses for a person or family. Financial planning is an important step for people with chronic medical conditions, such as Parkinson's disease [141, 143, 144, 147]

Flexible spending accounts: Accounts used to pay medical expenses not covered by insurance and that are set up through a person's employer [139]

Fludrocortisone: A corticosteroid used to manage neurogenic orthostatic hypotension [88, 89]

Freezing: An abrupt, uncontrolled stop in muscle movement that can happen to people with Parkinson's disease [24, 31, 123, 186]

Freezing of gait (FOG): The sudden inability to lift one's feet off the ground when walking, often while turning or changing directions or when attempting to do so; sometimes simply referred to as freezing [24, 30, 31, 123, 194]

APPENDIX C. Glossary & Index

Geriatrician: A primary care doctor who specializes in treating older individuals [119]

Globus pallidus: A structure located in the inner part of the basal ganglia that controls movement and can be affected by Parkinson's disease [74]

Hallucinate: To hear, feel, or smell something that is not real [29]

Hallucinations: Something that someone hears, feels, or smells that is not real [29, 32, 82, 83]

Health care proxy: A legal document in which a person has appointed an agent to make medical decisions in the event that the person is incapable of doing so [141]

Home health aide: A trained health care worker who provides patient assistance with personal care at home [140]

Human resources (HR): The personnel in a company who are responsible for hiring and training of employees, as well as administering employee benefits [135, 137, 194]

Hypomimia: Reduced facial expression; also known as facial masking, or more simply referred to as masking [32]

Impulse control disorder (ICD): Extreme changes in behavior such as gambling, excessive shopping, or hypersexuality [30, 84, 85, 194]

Infusion: Intravenous administration of medicine through a catheter or needle [72, 73]

Inner tremor: A tremor that is felt but not seen [25]

Insomnia: Sleep disorder characterized by having a hard time falling asleep, staying asleep, or both [32, 80, 81, 90, 92, 128, 151]

Involuntary rhythmic motion: Involuntary shaking of parts of the body such as hands; also known as tremor [23]

Istradefylline: An adenosine A_{2a} antagonist used to treat motor symptoms associated with Parkinson's disease by blocking a chemical in the brain called adenosine, an action that can reduce "off" periods

PD Keywords & Definitions

resulting from long-term treatment with levodopa. This medicine is used as an add-on treatment to carbidopa/levodopa [70]

Juvenile PD (JPD): Type of Parkinson's disease in children and teenagers whose onset of symptoms occurs before 21 years of age [19, 194]

Levodopa (L-dopa): A precursor of dopamine normally made by neurons. When dopamine-producing neurons degenerate, dopamine levels become low. Taking levodopa can effectively restore dopamine levels and improve mobility [several mentions, see table of contents]

Levodopa/carbidopa intestinal gel (LCIG) infusion: An alternative approach for the delivery of levodopa and carbidopa for individuals who are not managed well with traditional therapy. LCIG provides continuous infusion directly into the small intestine to reduce motor fluctuations and improve quality of life in advanced Parkinson's disease [72, 73, 194]

L-dopa: See Levodopa [Figures 3, 4, 7]

Long-term care insurance: An insurance policy to assist in paying for expenses related to long-term care [139, 140]

Magnetic resonance imaging (MRI): Medical imaging used to form pictures of the anatomy using strong magnetic fields [27, 195]

MAO-B inhibitors: Medicine that inhibits the activity of MAO-B enzymes and helps to preserve dopamine levels for people with Parkinson's disease [66, 68, 69, 70]

Medicaid: A federal- and state-level program that provides health coverage to low-income individuals [139, 145]

Medicare: A federal health insurance program for individuals over the age of 65 years [139, 140, 145]

Melvin Weinstein Parkinson's Foundation (MWPF): A nonprofit organization that provides medical equipment and supplies to individuals with Parkinson's disease to ensure a safe and healthy living environment (mwpf.org) [145, 195, 211]

APPENDIX C. Glossary & Index

The Michael J. Fox Foundation: A foundation committed to finding a cure for Parkinson's disease through research and development of therapies (michaeljfox.org) [11, 163, 173, 211]

Micrographia: A change in handwriting in which the writing becomes smaller or crowded due to difficulty with the fine motor movements that occurs with Parkinson's disease [28, 143, 144]

Midodrine: An alpha-adrenergic agonist used to treat symptoms associated with neurogenic orthostatic hypotension [88, 89]

Molecules: A collection of atoms that are bound together to form a single chemical unit [46]

Motor fluctuations: Pattern of "on" and "off" episodes when the levodopa level is sufficient and then insufficient for managing symptoms [59, 72, 73, 74]

Motor symptoms: The most common characteristic symptoms of Parkinson's disease, including slow movement, tightness, and stiffness of muscles, and a resting tremor. These symptoms usually start on one side of the body, then move to both sides
[several mentions, see table of contents]

Movement disorder specialists: Neurologists with additional training in movement disorders [26, 27, 105, 118, 195]

Multidisciplinary team: Health care team made up of different clinicians working together to manage a patient [118, 195]

Neurodegenerative condition: A debilitating condition that results in progressive degeneration of cells. Examples include Parkinson's and Alzheimer's disease [14]

Neurogenic orthostatic hypotension (NOH): A drop in blood pressure that occurs when standing up. It can also happen when going from lying down to sitting up, and can contribute to falls in people with Parkinson's disease [31, 88, 89, 195]

Neurologic: Refers to the nervous system and includes the brain, spine, cranial nerves, and peripheral nerves [3, 22, 86, 146]

Neurologist: A doctor specializing in brain conditions [26, 27, 118, 119, 172]

PD Keywords & Definitions

Neurons: Nerve cells [several mentions, see table of contents]

Neuropsychologist: A psychologist who specializes in understanding the relationship between the brain and behaviors [77]

Neurotransmitter: A specialized chemical produced in nerve cells that permits the transmission of information between cells (for example, dopamine) [3, 14, 44, 45, 66, 68, 71]

Nocturia: Excessive urination at night [33, 90, 95]

Non-motor symptoms: Symptoms that do not involve movement such as trouble multitasking, blood pressure fluctuations, or episodes of anxiety or excessive sweating; also known as invisible symptoms [several mentions, see table of contents]

Norepinephrine: A chemical neurotransmitter (found in the brain) [76, 78]

Occupational therapist: A health care professional who can identify ways to help you continue to do activities that are important to you. [77, 119, 191, 195]

"Off" episodes: Part of the motor fluctuations in which the level of levodopa is insufficient to control symptoms [59, 60, 63, 64, 66, 68, 70, 72, 75, 98]

"On" episodes: Part of the motor fluctuations in which the level of levodopa is sufficient to control symptoms [59, 60, 64, 66, 73]

Opicapone: A COMT inhibitor used to treat Parkinson's disease [68]

Overstimulation: When too much dopamine is present for a brief period of time "at the peak" causing uncontrollable "wiggly" or dance-like movements in the body [62]

Pallidotomy: A surgical procedure in which a tiny area of the globus pallidus is destroyed to help improve symptoms of Parkinson's disease [74]

Parkinson's disease psychosis (PDP): Behavior in people with advanced Parkinson's disease that includes hallucinations, delusions, or combination of both [29, 82, 195]

APPENDIX C. Glossary & Index

Parkinson's Foundation: A national organization dedicated to improving the care of individuals with Parkinson's disease and advance research to find a cure (parkinson.org) [52, 118, 124, 150, 152, 163, 211]

Parkinson's Foundation Caregiver Self-Assessment: Developed by the Parkinson's Foundation, this 12-item questionnaire assesses a caregiver's risk factors and needs in caring for a loved one [150]

Parkinson's Foundation Helpline [800-4PD-INFO (473-4636)]: The foundation's helpline staffed with health care professionals who can provide information on the symptoms and management of the disease, care, emotional support, and referrals to other resources [152]

Parkinson's IQ + You: A series of free in-person and virtual events from The Michael J. Fox Foundation designed to empower patients and care partners to manage the disease, learn about the latest research, and connect with local resources (michaeljfox.org/PDIQ) [163]

Parkinson's Passport: An information booklet for people with Parkinson's disease that includes their medicine and treatment information that can be carried when traveling [131, 132]

PD: Abbreviation for Parkinson's disease (for example, *The PD Companion*) [appears throughout]

Peak-dose dyskinesia: Uncontrollable "wiggly" or dance-like movements that may occur in the body of a person with Parkinson's disease approximately 60 to 90 minutes after taking a large amount of levodopa medicine [62, 71]

Peak level: Maximum level of levodopa in the bloodstream; from this point, levels slowly decline over time as levodopa is naturally eliminated from the body [59]

Personal health literacy: The degree to which individuals have the ability to find, understand, and use information and services to inform their health-related decisions and decide actions for themselves and others. Parkinson's disease health literacy refers to gaining greater knowledge and understanding of Parkinson's disease [9, 42, 43, 108, 111, 148, 160, 161, 162]

Pharmacist: A health care professional who prepares and dispenses prescriptions [119, 157]

Physiotherapist: A specialist who helps people with injuries, disabilities, or illness regain as much functional ability as possible [119, 195]

PD Keywords & Definitions

Podiatrist: A doctor who specializes in treating feet [119]

Positivity: The practice of having an optimistic attitude [105, 106, 149]

Postural instability: Difficulty with balance [24, 195]

Postural reflexes: Reflexes that keep the body upright and aligned [31]

Power of attorney: A legal document that gives a person authorization to act on behalf of someone who becomes incapacitated [141, 142]

Pramipexole: A dopamine agonist used to treat symptoms of Parkinson's disease [64]

Precision medicine: Management and tailoring of treatment to the unique causes of a disease in each person [3, 10, 17, 21]

Primer: A traditional, time-proven way to teach complex subjects using simple terms and examples, clear writing, and imagery. The goal is to educate effectively without overwhelming a person [43]

Pseudobulbar affect (PBA): Uncontrollable laughter or crying that occurs in some people with Parkinson's disease [30, 86, 87, 195]

Rasagiline: A MAO inhibitor used to treat Parkinson's disease [66]

Resting tremor: An involuntary rhythmic motion that disappears with movement, considered to be a motor symptom in people with Parkinson's disease [3, 10, 23, 25]

Rigidity: Tightness and stiffness in the limbs that is considered to be a motor symptom in a person with Parkinson's disease [23, 74, 99, 109, 195]

Ropinirole: A dopamine agonist used to treat symptoms of Parkinson's disease [64]

Rotigotine: A dopamine agonist in the form of a transdermal patch that is used to treat symptoms of Parkinson's disease [64]

Safinamide: A MAO inhibitor used to treat Parkinson's disease [66]

Selegiline: A MAO inhibitor used to treat Parkinson's disease [66]

APPENDIX C. Glossary & Index

Serotonin: A chemical neurotransmitter involved in regulating mood, energy, motivation, appetite, and sleep [78]

Sex therapist: A health professional who helps individuals and couples with sexual problems [119]

Shaking palsy: Old term that was used to refer to what is now Parkinson's disease [26]

Sialorrhea: Excessive drooling [33, 98, 99]

Side effects: An undesirable effect(s) of a medicine or other medical treatment or therapy [33, 54, 56, 59, 71, 73, 74, 75, 78, 82, 83, 90, 93, 100, 154]

Signals: An electric impulse or chemical process used to move information from one nerve cell to the next [several mentions, see table of contents]

Signal transmission: The movement of electric signals along a neuron, or chemical signals across a synapse [44, 45, 46, 86, 96]

Sleep-wake cycle: The pattern of time spent awake and asleep over 24 hours [90]

Social worker: A professional who helps individuals and communities meet basic and complex needs and enhance overall well-being [85, 119, 155]

Speech-language therapist: A specialist who helps treat difficulties associated with language, speech, and cognitive communication [99, 119]

Stooped: Change in posture that causes the head and shoulders to bend forward, potentially causing a person with Parkinson's disease to fall [31, 123]

Substantia nigra: Region of the brain that is involved with the control of muscle movement. Dopamine is an important neurotransmitter in this area of the brain [14, 15, 17, 44, 45, 47, 48, 52, 53, 62, 68]

Synapse: The space between 2 nerve cells [44, 45, 46, 48, 49]

Team-based approach: An approach in which different types of experts work with an individual on an as-needed basis to address the full range of symptoms [52]

PD Keywords & Definitions

Telecommuting: The practice of working remotely from home by using a computer and telephone [135]

The Parkinson Alliance: An organization that fundraises to support the development of new treatments and to find a cure for Parkinson's disease (parkinsonalliance.org) [163, 211]

Thermodysregulation: The inability to tolerate heat or cold temperatures, common in people with Parkinson's disease [126]

Titration: Slow increase or decrease of medicine dose over time [54]

Tolcapone: A COMT inhibitor used to treat Parkinson's disease [68]

Tremor: Involuntary movement of parts of the body that is associated with Parkinson's disease [several mentions, see table of contents]

Triggers: Events or exposure to toxins that can happen decades before symptoms develop. Most people exposed to these triggers will never develop Parkinson's disease because they don't have a facilitator [20, 21, 82, 86]

Tyrosine: An amino acid used by neurons to make dopamine [47, 48, 49, 53, 54]

Urinary tract infection: An infection caused by bacteria in the urinary system [95]

Urologist: A doctor who specializes in the treatment of disorders of the urinary system [95, 119]

Vivid dreams: Dreams that can be very intense and clear, but may also be disturbing making it difficult to sleep [90]

"Wearing-off" effect: The tendency, after receiving long-term levodopa treatment, for each dose of the drug to be effective for shorter episodes of time [60]

Well Spouse Association (WSA): A nonprofit organization that provides support to spouses of individuals who are ill or disabled (wellspouse.org) [163, 195, 211]

Will: A legal document that outlines a person's wishes on how to distribute their wealth and property, and who will care for minor children, after their death [141, 142]

Life With **PARKINSON'S**

APPENDIX D. Index to Key Figures

Figure 1: Signal Transmissions Moving ALONG 2 Nerve Cells and BETWEEN Cells Via Chemical Transmission 45

Figure 2: Tyrosine and Levodopa Crossing the Blood-Brain Barrier 47

Figure 3: Important Steps for Making New Dopamine, Storage, and Release by Nerve Cells 48

Figure 4: Dopamine Supply in the Brain Is a Balance Between New Dopamine Production and Dopamine Breakdown. 49

Figure 5: The Balance Between New Dopamine and Dopamine Breakdown Regulates Amount of Dopamine Available For Communication Between Nerve Cells. 50

Figure 6: Less New Dopamine Leads to Low Dopamine Supply 51

Figure 7: Adding Levodopa Can Increase Available Supply of Dopamine in Individuals With Parkinson's Disease 54

Figure 8: Taking Levodopa Can Increase Dopamine Levels In Parkinson's Disease. 55

Figure 9: Amount of Medicine in Blood Over Time, After Taking Each Dose of Levodopa by Mouth 59

Figure 10: Dopamine Agonists Can Substitute for Dopamine and Increase Supply in People With Parkinson's Disease 65

Figure 11: MAO-B Inhibitors Help Maintain Dopamine Supply 66

Figure 12: COMT Inhibitors Help Maintain Dopamine Supply 68

Figure 13: Balancing Act Between Dopamine (DA) and Acetylcholine (ACh) Can Influence Motor Symptoms 71

APPENDIX E. Parkinson's Resources

AMERICAN PARKINSON DISEASE ASSOCIATION
apdaparkinson.org

THE BRAIN INITIATIVE
braininitiative.nih.gov

CAREGIVER ACTION NETWORK (CAN)
caregiveraction.org

DAVIS PHINNEY FOUNDATION FOR PARKINSON'S
davisphinneyfoundation.org

THE EUROPEAN PARKINSON'S DISEASE ASSOCIATION
epda.eu.com

FAMILY CAREGIVER ALLIANCE (FCA)
caregiver.org

FOX TRIAL FINDER AT THE MICHAEL J. FOX FOUNDATION
michaeljfox.org/trial-finder

JOURNEY WITH PARKINSON'S
journeywithparkinsons.com

THE MELVIN WEINSTEIN PARKINSON'S FOUNDATION
mwpf.org

THE MICHAEL J. FOX FOUNDATION
michaeljfox.org

NATIONAL INSTITUTE OF NEUROLOGICAL DISEASES AND STROKE (NINDS)
ninds.nih.gov/Disorders/All-Disorders/Parkinsons-Disease-Information-Page

THE PARKINSON ALLIANCE
parkinsonalliance.org

PARKINSON SUPPORT & WELLNESS (PSW)
parkinsoncincinnati.org

PARKINSON'S FOUNDATION
parkinson.org

WELL SPOUSE ASSOCIATION
wellspouse.org

APPENDIX F. References

The following references were consulted during the development of **The PD Companion**.

American Parkinson Disease Association
apdaparkinson.org

Armstrong MJ, Okun MS. Diagnosis and treatment of Parkinson disease: a review. *JAMA*. 2020;323(6): 548-560.

Chen JJ, Dashitipour K. Parkinson's disease. In: *Pharmacotherapy: A Pathophysiologic Approach*. JT Dipiro, GC Lee, LM Posey, ST Haines, TD Holin, V Ellingrod, eds. New York, NY: McGraw Hill; 2020.

Davis Phinney Foundation For Parkinson's
davisphinneyfoundation.org

The European Parkinson's Disease Association
epda.eu.com

Hayes MT. Parkinson's disease and parkinsonism. *Am J Med*. 2019;132(7):802-807.

Homayoun H. Parkinson disease. *Ann Intern Med*. 2018; 169(5): ITC33-ITC48.

Jankovic J, Tan EK. Parkinson's disease: etiopathogenesis and treatment. *J Neurol Neurosurg Psychiatry*. 2020;91(8): 795-808.

Johnson ME, Stecher B, Labrie V, et al. Triggers, facilitators, and aggravators: redefining Parkinson's disease pathogenesis. *Trends Neurosci*. 2019;42(1):4-13.

Journey With Parkinson's
journeywithparkinsons.com

Parkinson's Foundation. *Medications; a treatment guide to Parkinson's disease*. Miami, FL: 2020.

The Melvin Weinstein Parkinson's Foundation
mwpf.org

The Michael J. Fox Foundation
michaeljfox.org

National Institute of Neurological Diseases and Stroke (NINDS)
ninds.nih.gov/Disorders/All-Disorders/Parkinsons-Disease-Information-Page

The Parkinson Alliance
parkinsonalliance.org

Parkinson Support & Wellness (PSW)
parkinsoncincinnati.org

Stoker TB, Greenland JC, eds. *Parkinson's Disease, Pathogenesis and Clinical Aspects*. Brisbane, Australia: Codon Publications; 2018.

Parkinson's Foundation
parkinson.org

Well Spouse Association
wellspouse.org